Treat Concussion, TBI, and PTSD with Vitamins and Antioxidants

Treat Concussion, TBI, and PTSD with Vitamins and Antioxidants

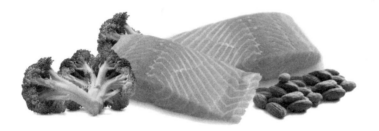

Kedar N. Prasad, Ph.D.

Healing Arts Press
Rochester, Vermont • Toronto, Canada

Healing Arts Press
One Park Street
Rochester, Vermont 05767
www.HealingArtsPress.com

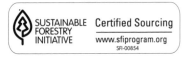

Text stock is SFI certified

Healing Arts Press is a division of Inner Traditions International

Note to the reader: *This book is intended as an informational guide. The remedies, approaches, and techniques described herein are meant to supplement, and not to be a substitute for, professional medical care or treatment. They should not be used to treat a serious ailment without prior consultation with a qualified health care professional.*

Library of Congress Cataloging-in-Publication Data

Prasad, Kedar N.
  Treat concussion, TBI, and PTSD with vitamins and antioxidants / Kedar N. Prasad, Ph.D.
    pages cm
  Includes bibliographical references and index.
  ISBN 978-1-62055-435-7 (paperback) — ISBN 978-1-62055-436-4 (e-book)
  1. Vitamin therapy. 2. Brain—Concussion. 3. Brain—Wounds and injuries—Alternative treatment. 4. Post-traumatic stress disorder—Alternative treatment. I. Title.
  RM259.P73 2016
  615.3'28—dc23

2015015201

Printed and bound in the United States by Lake Book Manufacturing, Inc. The text stock is SFI certified. The Sustainable Forestry Initiative® program promotes sustainable forest management.

10 9 8 7 6 5 4 3 2 1

Text design and layout by Virginia Scott Bowman
This book was typeset in Garamond Premier Pro and Gill Sans with Avant Garde and Helvetica Neue used as display typefaces

To send correspondence to the author of this book, mail a first-class letter to the author c/o Inner Traditions • Bear & Company, One Park Street, Rochester, VT 05767, and we will forward the communication, or contact the author directly at **knprasad@comcast.net.**

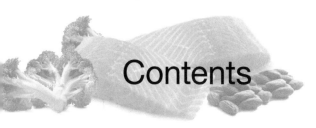

Contents

Foreword

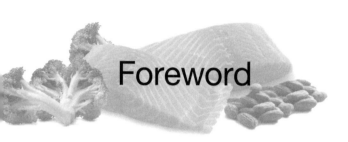

Physical injury to the brain is widespread and can have many causes. Vehicular accidents, domestic violence, and sports injuries can lead to serious brain injury in otherwise healthy young people. In combat zones, concussive brain injuries can lead to prolonged post-traumatic stress disorder. In addition to any acute injury to the brain, extended adverse consequences are a common feature.

The novel concept that Kedar Prasad has originated and presents in this book is that this long period of disruption of brain function following physical trauma also gives the opportunity for therapeutic intervention. He has developed a logical regimen incorporating many recent findings relevant to effecting restoration of optimal functioning by the brain. His approach is essentially nutritional and is inexpensive, non-invasive, and devoid of adverse toxic side effects. The plan that Prasad has designed has been found of broad applicability in several other disease states. This volume assembles the reasons validating each component of his design and explains the advantages of dietary supplementation with of a mixture of several kinds of probiotic agents.

This book is designed to be useful to a broad range of readers, and the material within it is readily accessible to non-scientists. The book will be especially valuable to physicians and other health care workers engaged in the care and treatment of victims of traumatic brain injury.

Modern medicine has allowed an increasing number of victims to survive the immediate consequences of brain injury, making the material in this report particularly relevant and an especially important contribution to current medical issues.

STEPHEN BONDY, PH.D.

Stephen Bondy, Ph.D., is a Professor of Neuroscience in the Center for Occupational and Environmental Health, University of California, Irvine. He obtained an M.A. from Cambridge University and a Ph.D. in Biochemistry from the University of Birmingham, UK. He has held positions at Columbia University, UCLA, University of Colorado, and the National Institute for Environmental Health Sciences. He is the author of over 300 articles and reviews. His earlier work included contributions to the relation between sensory input and brain energy metabolism, the factors influencing neurotransmitter receptor density, and the role of free radicals in neurotoxic damage.

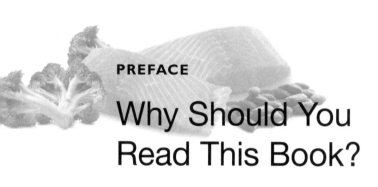

Why Should You Read This Book?

Although many neurological diseases exist to plague mankind, this book discusses only concussive injury, penetrating traumatic brain injury (penetrating TBI), and post-traumatic stress disorder (PTSD). These neurological abnormalities are induced by external agents, such as contact sports (concussive injury without fracture of the skull), accidents in which objects penetrate the skull (penetrating TBI), or explosive blasts or other extreme events that later lead to post-traumatic stress disorder (PTSD).

Among veterans of foreign wars, the incidence of PTSD and other mental disorders is being diagnosed at increased rates, which has become a major concern for the U.S. military. Among the veterans of Iraq and Afghanistan, the incidence of PTSD is about 18–20 percent; however, among the Vietnam veterans, the incidence of PTSD is about 31 percent in men and 27 percent in women. This suggests that the incidence rate among veterans of recent conflicts may increase in future. The incidence of TBI among American soldiers has risen from about 20 percent in the previous wars to 60 percent in the Iraq and Afghanistan conflicts.

Increasing numbers of high school, college, and professional athletes are participating in contact sports such as football, soccer, and ice hockey, and concussive injuries of the brain are being diagnosed on a more frequent basis among these individuals. It has been estimated that concussive injuries increased 4-fold between the years 1998 and 2008. Treatment of PTSD and TBI remain unsatisfactory and although physical protection against concussive injury and TBI exists, there is no adequate *biological* protection.

In this book, I propose a unified hypothesis: increased oxidative stress, chronic inflammation, and glutamate release are primarily responsible for the initiation and progression of concussive injury, penetrating TBI, and PTSD, because all of them are toxic to nerve cells. Additionally, I contend that imbalances between the action of excitatory neurotransmitter glutamate, and the inhibitory neurotransmitter gama-aminobutyric acid (GABA) result in increased activity of glutamate in the brain, which contributes to the progression of concussive injuries, penetrating TBI, and PTSD. Therefore, reducing oxidative stress, chronic inflammation, and glutamate release would appear to be one of the best choices for reducing the progression of the above-referenced neurological diseases.

This proposed micronutrient strategy in combination with standard therapy may improve the management of these neurological abnormalities more than that produced by standard therapy alone. In order to reduce oxidative stress, chronic inflammation, and glutamate release, it's essential to simultaneously increase the levels of all antioxidant enzymes and all dietary and endogenous antioxidants. (Endogenous antioxidants are those that are made by the body.) This goal cannot be achieved by the use of only one or two antioxidants. Therefore, I have proposed a preparation of micronutrients containing *multiple* dietary and endogenous antioxidants, vitamin D, selenium, B vitamins, and certain polyphenolic compounds (curcumin and resveratrol) and omega-3 fatty acids, for reducing the risk of the progression of the neurodegenerative conditions discussed in this book. These micronutrients are efficacious because they increase the levels of *all* antioxidant enzymes by activating a nuclear transcriptional factor-2/ antioxidant response element (Nrf2/ARE) pathway, as well as enhancing the levels of dietary and endogenous antioxidant chemicals.

Even though some laboratory data exists to suggest that even the genetic basis of neurological disease can be prevented or delayed by micronutrient supplements, the increase in the amount of micronutrients that I propose flies in the face of conventional theory, for most neurologists believe that antioxidants and vitamins have no significant role in the prevention or improved management of neurodegenerative diseases. These beliefs are primarily based on a few clinical studies in which supplementation with a single antioxidant, such as vitamin E in Alzheimer's disease or coenzyme Q10 in Parkinson's disease, produced only modest beneficial effects in the study group. Another study demonstrated that vitamin E alone was ineffective in reducing the progression of Parkinson's disease.

Although some books on neurodegenerative diseases and their causes and symptoms are available, none of them have critically analyzed the published data on antioxidant and neurodegenerative diseases, and have never questioned whether the experimental designs of the study on which the conclusions were based were scientifically valid, whether the results obtained from the use of a single antioxidant in high-risk population can be extrapolated to the effect of the same antioxidant in a multiple antioxidant preparation for the same population, and whether the results of studies obtained on high-risk populations can be extrapolated to normal populations.

The fact of the matter is that patients with neurodegenerative diseases may have a high oxidative environment in the brain, thus the administration of a single antioxidant *should not be expected* to produce any significant beneficial effects. This is due to the fact that an individual antioxidant in the presence of a high oxidative environment may be oxidized, and then act as a pro-oxidant rather than as an antioxidant. Also, the levels of the oxidized form of an antioxidant may increase after the prolonged consumption of a single antioxidant; this can subsequently damage brain cells. Coupled with this is the fact that a single antioxidant cannot elevate *all* antioxidant enzymes as well as a multitude of dietary and endogenous antioxidants.

I have published several reviews in peer-reviewed journals challenging the current trends of using single antioxidants in the prevention or improved management of neurodegenerative diseases in high-risk populations. These articles, however, have failed to have any significant impact on the design of clinical trials, and the inconsistent results of the effects of a single antioxidant continue to be published.

Be that as it may, there is increasing debate on this issue. These growing controversies regarding the value of multiple micronutrients in the prevention and improved management of neurodegenerative diseases need to be addressed and new solutions need to be proposed. Thus I advocate for an approach that supports the further study of multiple micronutrients in this medical context.

The rationale for using the proposed preparation of micronutrients in clinical studies on neurodegenerative diseases is supported by two recent clinical studies on other diseases. In contrast to previous studies in which supplementation with beta-carotene alone increased the risk of lung cancer among heavy tobacco smokers, two clinical studies with a preparation of *multiple* antioxidants *reduced* the incidence of cancer by 10 percent, and improved clinical outcomes in patients with HIV/AIDS. These studies were published in the *Journal of American Medical Association* (Gaziano et al. 2012, and Baum et al. 2013), a highly prestigious journal.

A comprehensive preparation of micronutrients containing multiple dietary and endogenous antioxidants, B vitamins, vitamin D, selenium, and certain polyphenolic compounds (curcumin and resveratrol) and omega-3 fatty acids for the prevention and/or improved management of neurodegenerative diseases in conjunction with standard therapy has never been proposed until now.

I hope that my work will serve as a guide to those individuals who are interested in using micronutrients to reduce the risk of the progression of the debilitating neurodegenerative diseases discussed in this book. Primary care physicians and practicing neurologists interested in complementary medicine may find this information useful in recommending micronutrient supplements to their patients.

Consumers who are taking daily supplements will find the information provided herein encouraging. Those who are not taking supplements or are uncertain as to their potential benefits may find evidence to help them make a decision as to whether or not to take micronutrient supplements daily, in consultation with their doctors.

ACKNOWLEDGMENTS

I would like to thank my family for their support and encouragement. I also am very thankful to Anne Dillon and Chanc VanWinkle Orzell for their superb editing of this book.

1 Structure and Function of the Human Brain

Despite extensive research by neuroanatomists, neurobiologists, neurochemists, and neurophysiologists, many aspects of the brain's structure and functioning remain tantalizingly unclear. The "Decade of the Brain," an initiative of the U.S. government in the 1990s under President George Bush, has increased our knowledge of brain functioning somewhat. Still, the work goes on to discover its myriad mysteries. Research endeavors include the study of animal and human neuronal and glial cell culture, the brain tissue of animals (primarily rodents and occasionally nonhuman primates), and human brains obtained at autopsy. Current research also includes noninvasive techniques such as electroencephalography (EEG), functional magnetic resonance imaging (fMRI), as well as invasive techniques such as obtaining fresh brain tissues from animals after euthanasia and human brain samples obtained whenever possible during surgery.

This chapter describes very briefly, and in simple terms, the structure and functions of the human brain that are relevant to chronic neurological diseases. It's important to have a fundamental understanding of how the brain works so that we can better understand the dynamics involved when it becomes impaired.

1

THE HUMAN BRAIN

Basic Facts

The average weight of the human adult brain is about three pounds (1.5 kilograms). In women the volume of the brain is approximately 1,130 cubic centimeters and in men it is about 1,260 cubic centimeters, although significant individual variations are found. The brain consists of three main regions: the forebrain, midbrain, and hindbrain. Brain regions are divided into the cerebrum, the cerebellum, the limbic system, and the brain stem.

The brain also contains four interconnected cavities that are filled with cerebrospinal fluid, as well as approximately 100 billion neurons. Neurons are a unique type of cell in that they can receive, synthesize, store, and transmit information from one neuron to another. Figure 1.1 presents a view of various structures of the human brain.

The Cerebrum and Its Function

The cerebrum or cortex is the largest part of the human brain, having a surface area of about 1.3 square feet (0.12 m2), folded in such a way so as to allow it to fit within the skull. This folding causes ridges of the cerebrum; these are called "gyri" collectively or "gyrus" in the singular. Crevices in the cortex are called "sulcus" or "sulci" (collectively). The cerebrum is divided into the right and left hemispheres, which are connected by a fibrous band of nerves called the corpus callosum. The corpus callosum is responsible for communication between the hemispheres. The right hemisphere controls the left side of the body and oversees temporal and spatial relationships, the analysis of nonverbal information, and the communication of emotion. The left hemisphere controls the right side of the body and produces and understands language.

The cortex of each hemisphere is divided into four lobes: the frontal lobe, the parietal lobe, the occipital lobe, and the temporal lobe. Certain functions of the lobes overlap with one another. The fron-

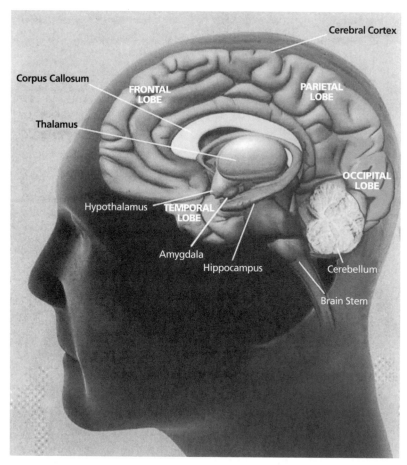

Figure 1.1. This image shows a horizontal slice of the head of an adult man, revealing the different structures of the human brain. Courtesy of the National Library of Medicine's Visible Human Project.

tal lobe is responsible for cognition and memory, behavior, abstract thought processes, problem solving, analytic and critical reasoning, attention, creative thought, voluntary motor activity, language skills, emotional traits, intellect, reflection, judgment, physical reaction, inhibition, libido (the sexual urge), and initiative.

The parietal lobe oversees basic sensations such as touch, pain, pressure, temperature sensitivity, various joint movements, tactile sensations, spatial relationships and sensitivity to an exact point of tactile contact, as well as the ability to distinguish between two points of tactile stimulation, some language and reading functions, and some visual functions.

The occipital lobe is involved in interpreting visual impulses and reading.

The temporal lobe is involved with auditory (sound) sensations, speech, the sensation of smell, one's sense of identity, fear, music, some hearing, some vision pathways, and some emotions and memories.

Nerve cells form the gray surface of the cerebrum, which is a little thicker than the nerve fibers that carry signals between nerve cells and other parts of the body.

The Cerebellum

The cerebellum is much smaller than the cerebrum, but like the cerebrum, it has a highly folded surface. This portion of the brain is associated with the coordination of movement; posture and balance; and cardiac, respiratory, and vasomotor functions.

The Limbic System

The limbic system includes the thalamus, hypothalamus, amygdala, and hippocampus. It is responsible for processing emotion and storing and retrieving memory.

The Thalamus

The thalamus is a large, paired, egg-shaped structure containing clusters of nuclei (gray matter); it is responsible for sensory and motor functions. Sensory information enters the thalamus, which relays the information to the overlying cerebral cortex.

The Hypothalamus

The hypothalamus is located ventral to the thalamus and is responsible for regulating emotion, thirst, hunger, circadian rhythms, the autonomic nervous system, and the pituitary gland.

The Amygdala

The amygdala is located in the temporal lobe just beneath the surface of the hippocampus and is associated with memory, emotion, and fear.

The Hippocampus

The hippocampus is that portion of the cerebral hemisphere in the basal medial part of the temporal lobe. It is responsible for learning and memory. It is also responsible for converting short-term memory to more permanent memory and for recalling spatial relationships.

The Brain Stem

The brain stem is located underneath the limbic system. It's responsible for regulating breathing, heartbeat, and blood pressure. The main constituents of the brain stem are the midbrain, pons, medulla, and the pyramidal and extrapyramidal systems.

The Midbrain

The midbrain, also called the mesencephalon, is located between the forebrain and the hindbrain (pons and medulla), and includes the tectum and the tegmentum. The midbrain participates in regulating motor functions, eye movements, pupil dilation, and hearing. The midbrain also contains the crus cerebri, which is made up of nerve fibers. These nerve fibers connect the cerebral hemispheres to the cerebellum and substantia nigra. The substantia nigra neurons are pigmented and consist of two parts, the pars reticulate and the pars compacta. Nerve cells of the pars compacta contain dark pigments (melanin granules). These neurons synthesize dopamine and project to either the caudate nucleus or the putamen. Both the caudate nucleus and the putamen are part of the basal ganglia, which regulate movement and coordination. The striatum part of the brain consists of the globus pallidus, the substantia nigra, and the basal ganglia.

The Pons

The pons (metencephalon) is located below the posterior portion of the cerebrum and above the medulla oblongata. It regulates arousal and sleep and participates in controlling autonomic functions. It also relays sensory information between the cerebrum and the cerebellum.

The Medulla (Medulla Oblongata)

The medulla, also called the myelencephalon, is the lower portion of the brain stem and is located anterior to the cerebellum. It regulates autonomic functions and relays nerve signals between the brain and the spinal cord.

The Pyramidal and Extrapyramidal Systems

Both the pyramidal and the extrapyramidal systems represent part of the motor pathways within the brain stem. Neurons of the pyramidal system have no synapses, whereas neurons of the extrapyramidal system have synapses. Nerve fibers of the pyramidal system originate in the cerebral cortex and continue on to the thalamus and medulla oblongata. The pyramidal system regulates fine movements such as control of the jaws, lips, and aspects of the face, conscious thoughts, and movements of the hands and fingers.

The major parts of the extrapyramidal system include the red nucleus, the caudate nucleus, the putamen, the substantia nigra, the globus pallidus, and the subthalamic nuclei. The extrapyramidal system dampens erratic motions, maintains muscle tone, and allows for overall functional stability.

Other Components of the Brain

Basal Ganglia

The basal ganglia is located deep in the cerebral hemisphere. It consists of the caudate nucleus, the putamen, the globus pallidus, the substantia nigra, and the subthalamic nucleus. It regulates posture and emotion, such as happiness, through dopamine. It also regulates movements and their intensity.

Neurons

Neurons (nerve cells) in the brain are highly complex, specialized cells that receive information, process it, and then send it in the form of electrical impulses through synapses to other neurons. (Synapses connect a neuron to other neurons.) A diagrammatic representation of a neuron is provided in figure 1.2. The estimation of the number of neurons in the brain varies from study to study, with one study estimating that the human brain contains about 100 billion neurons and about 100 trillion synapses (Williams and Herrup 1988). Approximately 3 to 5 percent of neurons are lost from the brain every decade after the age of thirty-five. Therefore, it's possible that older individuals may have fewer neurons than the aforementioned estimated 100 billion neurons.

A neuron consists of the cell body (also called soma), dendrites, and an axon. The cell body contains a nucleus, mitochondria, Golgi

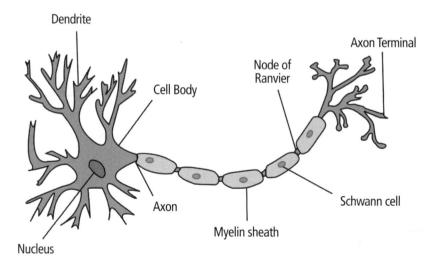

Figure 1.2. A typical neuron

bodies, and lysosomes, as well as smooth and rough endoplasmic reticulum. Dendrites are filamentous structures that extend away from the cell body. They branch into several processes that become thinner the further they extend. An axon is also a filamentous structure that extends itself from the cell body at a swelling called the axon hillock, which branches away from the soma. As it extends further it undergoes further branching at the axonal terminal. These branches, through synapses, can communicate with more than one neuron at a time.

The soma can have numerous dendrites, but only one axon. The axons of presynaptic neurons contain mitochondria and microtubules. The microtubules help to transport neurotransmitters from the cytoplasm to the tip of the axon where they're stored in very small vesicles. Incoming synaptic signals from other neurons are received by the dendrites; the outgoing signals are sent through the axons.

Presynaptic neurons are those that transmit signals to different neurons through the axon and its synapses. The neurons that receive these signals are called postsynaptic neurons. Axon terminals contain neurotransmitters that are released at the postsynaptic neurons.

There are three major specialized neurons: sensory neurons, motor neurons, and interneurons. Sensory neurons respond to touch, sound, light, and many other stimuli. They affect the cells of sensory organs and then send signals to the brain and the spinal cord. Motor neurons receive signals from the brain and the spinal cord, cause muscle contractions, and affect glands. Interneurons connect neurons to other neurons within the same regions of the brain.

Other neurons include cholinergic neurons, dopaminergic neurons, glutamatergic neurons, GABAergic neurons, and serotonergic neurons. They are described below.

Cholinergic neurons: Cholinergic neurons are primarily located in the basal forebrain, striatum, and cerebral cortex. Each neuron contains an enzyme choline acetyltransferase, which makes the neurotransmitter acetylcholine from choline. Acetylcholine is degraded by another enzyme called acetylcholinesterase. Acetylcholine is stored in small vesicles in the nerve endings. An elevation of extracellular calcium causes the release of acetylcholine from the vesicles. The action of this neurotransmitter is mediated through nicotinic receptors and muscarinic receptors. Cholinergic neurons are the primary source of acetylcholine for the cerebral cortex; acetylcholine regulates memory and learning ability.

Dopaminergic neurons: Dopamine belongs to the group of catecholamines. It is degraded by the enzyme catechol-O-methyltransferase (COMT). Neurons that produce dopamine (dopaminergic neurons) are also referred to as dopamine (DA) neurons. Dopaminergic neurons make a neurotransmitter dopamine (3,4-dihydroxyphenethylamine) from L-DOPA (L-3,4-dihydroxyphenylalanine) with the help of the enzyme DOPA decarboxylase. L-dopa is made from the amino acid tyrosine by the enzyme tyrosine hydroxylase. Dopamine neurons are primarily located in the substantia nigra pars compacta, a part of the basal ganglia present in the midbrain. This area of the brain also contains melanin granules and a high level of iron (Chinta and Andersen 2005). The presence of melanin granules and iron exposes dopamine neurons to increased levels of free radicals.

The ventral tegmental area of the midbrain also contains dopamine neurons, which send their projections to the striatum, globus pallidus, and subthalamic nucleus. Although the number of dopamine neurons is relatively less, they regulate several functions, including voluntary movement, mood reward addiction, stress, motivation, arousal, and sexual gratification. The action of dopamine is mediated via dopamine receptors D1-5. Dopamine is converted to norepinephrine by the enzyme dopamine B-carboxylase and norepinephrine is converted to epinephrine by the enzyme phenylethanolamine-N-methyltransferase.

Catecholamines (dopamine, norepinephrine, and epinephrine) are degraded by the enzyme COMT and/or monoamine oxidase.

Glutamatergic neurons: Neurons producing glutamate are called glutamatergic neurons. Glutamate is considered one of the most important neurotransmitters for proper brain functioning. As mentioned earlier it is considered excitatory because it causes hyperactivity and kills neurons by excitotoxicity. Excitotoxicity refers to the ability of glutamate to kill neurons by producing prolonged excitatory synaptic transmission. Glutamate mediates its actions through its receptors N-methyl-D-aspartate (NMDA), a-amino-3-hydroxy-5-methyl-4-isoxazolepropionic acid (AMPA), kianate, and G-protein coupled glutamate receptors (mGLuR1).

Glutamate is a nonessential amino acid that does not cross the blood-brain barrier. It is made in the neurons from glutamine that is present in the synaptic terminal. Glutamine is released from glial cells and accumulates in the presynaptic terminal where it is converted to glutamate by the mitochondrial enzyme glutaminase. Glutamate is stored in very small vesicles and is released from these vesicles by the glutamate transporters present in glial cells and presynaptic terminals. Glutamate is converted back to glutamine by the enzyme glutamine synthetase, which is present in glial cells. Glutamine is then transported from the glial cells to presynaptic nerve terminals.

More than half of the brain synapses release glutamate. Following brain injury, glutamate is released and accumulates in the extracellular space of the brain. This is responsible for the neurodegeneration that is commonly found in some neurodegenerative diseases. An increase in the extracellular levels of glutamate in the brain is associated with some neurological conditions, such as concussive injury, traumatic brain injury, post-traumatic stress disorder (PTSD), and Huntington's disease.

GABAergic neurons: Neurons producing gamma-aminobutyric acid (GABA) are called GABAergic neurons. As opposed to the excitatory function of glutamate, GABA exhibits inhibitory transmission and thereby balances the effect of glutamate on the neurons. It's been estimated that about 25 percent of neurons in the cortex use GABA (Tamminga et al. 2004). Like glutamate, GABA does not cross the blood-brain barrier. It is made in the neuron from glutamate by the enzyme L-glutamic acid decarboxylase and converted back to glutamate by a metabolic process called GABA shunt. The first step in the GABA shunt is to convert α-ketoglutarate into L-glutamic acid by the enzyme GABA α-oxoglutarate transaminase. Glutamic acid decarboxylase (GAD) converts glutamic acid into GABA.

Like glutamate, GABA is a nonessential amino acid. It mediates its action through GABA receptors (GABAa and GABAb). GABAa receptors regulate rapid mood changes as well as fear and anxiety. These receptors are the target for sedative drugs such as alcohol, benzodiazepines, and barbiturates. GABAb receptors regulate memory and depressed moods and pain. Stimulation of this receptor can reduce the release of dopamine that would inhibit the reward response induced by external agents such recreational drugs.

Purkinje neurons: Purkinje neurons are the largest neurons; they belong to the class of GABA neurons that are located in the cortex of the cerebellum. They can have over 1,000 dendritic branches. One Purkinje neuron can make connections with several neurons. These neurons possess a bidirectional signaling axis, which produces inhibitory as well as excitatory interneurons that play an important role in motor learning and general learning ability (Fleming et al. 2013).

Serotonergic neurons: Neurons producing serotonin (5-HT) are called serotonergic neurons. Serotonergic neurons are located in the raphe nuclei of the midbrain, pons, and medulla; they also accumulate in the synaptic clefts. The levels of serotonin in the synaptic cleft depend on the synthesis as well as the reuptake of serotonin. Serotonin neurons send projections to the cortex and basal ganglia.

Serotonin (5-hydroxytryptamine) is made from the amino acid tryptophan by the enzymes tryptophan hydroxylase and tryptophan decarboxylase. Serotonin does not cross the blood-brain barrier, however, L-tryptophan and its metabolite 5-hydroxytryptophan can enter the blood-brain barrier and increase the brain's level of serotonin. Serotonin mediates its action through serotonin receptors (5HT-1 and 5HT-2). It regulates mood, appetite, sleep, and, to some extent, memory and learning ability.

Glial Cells

Glial cells are totally different from nerve cells. Characterized by the presence of glial fibrillary acidic protein (GFAP), which is specific to them, they're considered supporting cells for the development, survival, and synaptic functions of neurons. They also help in the repair processes after an injury to the brain. Like neurons, they don't divide in the adult brain, but unlike neurons, they rapidly divide in response to brain injury. They do not have axons or elaborate neurites. The number of glial cells in the brain is much higher than the number of nerve cells. Indeed, the glial cells' main role is to support the nerve cells and to ensure their proper functioning. (The term "glial" is derived from the Greek word for "glue.") There are three types of glial cells in mature human brains: astrocytes, oligodendrocytes, and microglia cells.

Astrocytes: Astrocytes have small cytoplasmic processes that give an appearance of stars. They remove excess neurotransmitters released from nerve terminals and thereby regulate synaptic transmission. These cells also help to maintain concentrations of calcium and potassium in the brain.

Oligodendrocytes: Oligodendrocytes produce myelin, which wraps around the axons of neurons. The myelin sheath of oligodendrocytes forms electrical insulation around the nerve fibers and thereby facilitates rapid transmission of electrical signals in the brain.

Microglia: Microglia cells are smaller in size and are considered immune cells of the brain. In response to cellular injury the microglia migrate to the site of injury to help in the healing processes. These cells also produce pro-inflammatory cytokines that can damage neurons if the injury persists.

Growth Factors

Brains produce growth factors, which include nerve growth factor (NGF), brain-derived neurotrophic factor (BDNF), and glial cell-derived neurotrophic factor (GDNF). These growth factors are important in the development, survival, and regeneration of neurons following an injury. Both astrocytes and embryonic neurons from the mouse brain produce nerve growth factor in culture. The levels of nerve growth factor were higher in the growth phase than in the nongrowth phase. Unlike astrocytes, embryonic neurons continue to produce nerve growth factor during the nongrowth phase (Houlgatte et al. 1989).

It has been demonstrated that the presence of both glial cell-derived neurotrophic factor and brain-derived neurotrophic factor is required for the survival of certain neurons, including dopamine neurons (Erickson, Brosenitsch, and Katz 2001).

Brain-derived neurotrophic factors act via their respective receptors.

In a clinical study of 91 teenagers, it was demonstrated that serum levels of brain-derived neurotrophic factor increased after exercise and improved cognitive function (Lee et al. 2014). The level of basic fibroblastic growth factor (bFGF) increases in glioma cells. It has been demonstrated that insertion of basic fibroblastic growth factor into astrocytes causes a migration and proliferation of cells without tumor formation (Holland and Varmus 1998).

This observation suggests that increased levels of basic fibroblastic growth factor are not related to cancer formation in glial cells. An elevation of basic fibroblastic growth factor may be a signal for the astrocytes to divide.

Neurotransmitters

Neurotransmitters are chemicals produced in the neurons and are located primarily at the synapses. They carry signals from one neuron to another; these signals may be inhibitory or excitatory. Neurotransmitters are released in response to a specific stimulus; all have different functions. Electric charges from the cytoplasm of the neurons release neurotransmitters and send them across the synapse. They travel through the gap junction to bind with the receptors specific to a particular neurotransmitter located on the surface of postsynaptic neurons.

Synapses

A synapse is the junction between two neurons (presynaptic neurons and postsynaptic neurons). The gap between two neurons is about 0.02 microns.

Processes of the Brain

Conduction of Signals

In order to communicate neurons send electrical signals (action potential) to other neurons through the axons. This process of sending electrical signals is called conduction. An electrical signal is formed when ions, which are electrically charged particles, move across the neuronal membrane. The movement of ions takes place through ion channels that can open or close in the presence of neurotransmitters. The neuronal membrane is normally at rest (in a polarized state). The influx and outflux of ions through ion channels during neurotransmission depolarizes the target neuron. When this depolarization reaches a point of no return (threshold), a large electrical signal is generated. This electrical signal propagates along the axon until it reaches the axon terminal where the conduction of the electrical signal ends. The neuron then sends its output to other neurons.

Synaptic Transmission (Neurotransmission)

Synaptic transmission between neurons occurs by the movement of an electric or chemical signal across a synapse. At the electrical synapse the electrical signals are considered output, whereas at the chemical synapse neurotransmitters are considered output. At the electrical synapses two neurons are physically connected to each other through the gap junction that we mentioned earlier. The gap junction allows changes in the electrical signal of one neuron to affect the other. Chemical synaptic neurotransmission occurs at the chemical synapse. In this type of transmission the presynaptic neurons and the postsynaptic neurons are separated by the synaptic cleft. The synaptic cleft allows signals coming from one neuron to pass to another neuron.

CONCLUDING REMARKS

The human brain is the body's most complex organ about which much is still unknown. It's composed of approximately 100 billion neurons and 100 trillion synapses that extend over three areas: the forebrain, midbrain, and hindbrain. Parts of the brain include the cerebrum, the cerebellum, the limbic system, and the brain stem. Four cavities filled with cerebrospinal fluid are also part of the brain.

Brain cells include the neurons mentioned above, as well as glial cells. Neurons, both presynaptic and postsynaptic, hold and transmit information via the synapses in a process known as conduction. There are many different types of brain neurons; each type has a different function. Chemicals that transport signals from neuron to neuron, called neurotransmitters, are also part of the picture. Glial cells support the neurons and help to heal the brain in the case of brain injury. Substances called "growth factors" are produced by the brain and help neurons to recover following brain injury.

Now that we have discussed the components of the brain, its structure, and how it functions, let's turn our attention to the overall functioning of the human body in terms of how it relates to different types of stress, infection, and injury, and how the immune system attempts to protect it in the face of these stressors.

2 Oxidative Stress, Inflammation, and the Immune System

INTRODUCTION

This chapter describes oxidative stress caused by free radicals, types and sources of free radicals, inflammation, and the immune system briefly and in general terms.* These issues are huge and complex but herein we have attempted to describe them simply so that they may be easily grasped. A basic understanding of these biological processes and agents is essential for developing improved management strategies for the debilitating neurological symptoms of concussive injury, penetrating traumatic brain injury, and post-traumatic stress disorder.

WHAT IS OXIDATIVE STRESS?

Oxidative stress is a process that occurs when free radicals overwhelm the protective antioxidant systems of the body. What are

---

*Some of the references and books that have been used to prepare this chapter are Cotran 1999; Ryter 1985; Langermans, Hazenbos, and van Furth 1994; Holtmeier and Kabelitz 2005; Sproul et al. 2000; Kehry and Hodgkin 1994; Asmus 1994; Vaillancourt et al. 2008; Pryor 1994; Kehrer 1994.

free radicals? They are atoms, molecules, or ions with unpaired electrons—derived from either oxygen or nitrogen—which makes them highly reactive. However, although they can damage cells, they also play an important role in the regulation of certain bio-chemical processes and gene expressions necessary for our survival. In 1900 the first organic free radical, triphenylmethyl radical, was identified by Moses Gomberg of the University of Michigan. Free radicals are symbolized by a dot "•".

The half-lives of various free radicals vary from 10^{-9} seconds to days. This means most are quickly destroyed after causing damage. For example, the half-life of hydroxyl free radicals is 10^{-9} seconds, superoxide anion 10^{-5} seconds, lipid peroxyl free radical 7 seconds, semiquinone free radical days, nitric oxide about 1 second, and hydrogen peroxide minutes. The half-lives of some organic free radi-cals are several days.

TYPES OF FREE RADICALS

There are several different types of free radicals derived from oxy-gen and nitrogen that are generated in the body. The oxygen-derived free radicals include hydroxyl radical (OH•), peroxyl radical (ROO•), alkoxyl radical (RO•), phenoxyl and semiquinone radicals (ArO•, HO-Ar-O•), and superoxide radical ($O^{•-}_2$). The nitrogen-derived free radicals include NO, •ONOO$^-$ (peroxynitrite), and •NO$_2$.

SOURCES OF FREE RADICALS

Normally, free radicals are generated in the body during the use of oxy-gen in the metabolism of certain compounds. Mitochondria, which are elongated membranous structures present in all cells in varying num-bers, use oxygen to produce energy. During the process of generating energy, superoxide anions, hydroxyl radicals, and hydrogen peroxide are produced as by-products. It is estimated that about 2 percent of the oxygen consumed by the mitochondria remains partially used, and this unused oxygen leaks out of the mitochondria to make approximately 20 billion molecules of superoxide anions and hydrogen peroxide per cell per day.

During bacterial or viral infection, phagocytic cells are activated, generating high levels of nitric oxide superoxide anions and hydrogen peroxide within the infected cells in order to kill infective agents. Excessive production of free radicals by phagocytes can also damage normal cells, thereby increasing the risk of acute and/or chronic disease.

During the oxidative metabolism of fatty acids and other molecules in the body, free radicals are produced. Certain habits such as tobacco smoking, and the presence of some trace minerals such as free iron, copper, and manganese, can also increase the rate of production of free radicals. Thus is the human body exposed daily to different types and varying levels of free radicals.

OXIDATION AND
REDUCTION PROCESSES

To more fully understand the role that free radicals play, it's beneficial to grasp the relationship between the processes of oxidation and reduction that are constantly taking place in the body.

Oxidation is a process by which an atom or a molecule gains oxygen, loses hydrogen, or loses an electron. For example, carbon gains oxygen during oxidation and becomes carbon dioxide. A superoxide radical loses an electron during the oxidation process and becomes oxygen. Thus, an *oxidizing agent* is an atom or molecule that changes another chemical by adding oxygen to it or by removing an electron or hydrogen from it. Examples of oxidizing agents include free radicals, X-rays, and ozone.

Other oxidizing agents formed in the body include peroxynitrite, hydrogen peroxide, and lipid peroxide, all of which are very damaging to the cells. Many other radical species can be formed by biological reactions. These include phenolic and other aromatic compounds that are formed during metabolism of xenobiotic agents (agents that are foreign to the body).

Reduction is a process by which an atom or molecule loses oxygen, gains hydrogen, or gains an electron. For example, carbon dioxide loses oxygen and becomes carbon monoxide, carbon gains hydrogen and becomes methane, and oxygen gains an electron and becomes a superoxide anion. Thus, a *reducing agent* is an atom or molecule that changes another chemical by removing oxygen from it or by adding an electron or hydrogen to it.

All antioxidants may be considered reducing agents. Increased reduction processes over oxidation processes maintain cells in a healthy state, however, increased oxidation processes over reduction processes can lead to cellular injury, and eventually to chronic neurodegenerative diseases.

As we have learned, oxidative stress occurs when the generation of reactive oxygen species exceeds the antioxidant defense system's ability to neutralize them. Similarly, nitrosylative stress occurs when the generation of reactive nitrogen species exceeds the antioxidant defense system's ability to neutralize them. A chronic increase in oxidative and nitrosylative stress has been implicated in the initiation and progression of most human chronic diseases. However, short-term increased oxidative stress such as is seen during viral or bacterial infection may be important in killing invading organisms (although it can also damage normal tissue). Free radicals can damage DNA (deoxyribonucleic acid), RNA (ribonucleic acid), proteins, carbohydrates, and membranes.

The Formation of Free Radicals Derived
from Oxygen and Nitrogen

The formative process of some reactive oxygen species (ROS: free radicals derived from oxygen) is described below.

When molecular oxygen (O_2) acquires an electron, the superoxide anion ($O_2{}^{\bullet-}$) is formed:

$$O_2 + e^- = O_2{}^{\bullet-}$$

Superoxide dismutase (SOD) and H^+ can react with $O_2{}^{\bullet-}$ to form hydrogen peroxide (H_2O_2):

$$2O_2{}^{\bullet-} + 2H^+ \text{ plus SOD} \rightarrow H_2O_2 + O_2$$
$$O_2{}^{\bullet-} + H^+ \rightarrow HO_2{}^{\bullet} \text{ (hydroperoxy radical)}$$
$$2HO_2{}^{\bullet} \rightarrow H_2O_2 + O_2$$

Ferric and ferrous forms of iron can react with superoxide anion and hydrogen peroxide to produce molecular oxygen (O_2) and hydroxyl radicals ($OH^{\bullet}$), respectively:

$$Fe^{3+} + O_2{}^{\bullet-} \rightarrow Fe^{2+} + O_2$$
$$Fe_2{}^+ + H_2O_2 \rightarrow Fe^{3+} + OH^{\bullet} + OH^- \text{ (Fenton reaction)}$$

Hydroxyl radicals can also be formed from superoxide anion by the Haber-Weiss reaction:

$$O_2{}^{\bullet-} + H_2O_2 \rightarrow O_2 + OH^- + OH^{\bullet}$$

Both the Fenton and Haber-Weiss reactions require a transition metal such as copper or iron. Among ROS, $OH^{\bullet}$ is the most damaging free radical and is very short-lived.

Hydroxyl radicals are very reactive with a variety of organic compounds, leading to the production of more radical compounds:

$$RH \text{ (organic compound)} + OH^{\bullet} \rightarrow R^{\bullet} \text{ (organic radical)} + H_2O$$
$$R^{\bullet} + O_2 \rightarrow RO_2{}^{\bullet} \text{ (peroxyl radical)}$$

For example, the DNA radical can be generated by reaction with a hydroxyl radical, and this can lead to a break in the DNA strand.

Catalase detoxifies hydrogen peroxide to form water and molecular oxygen:

$$H_2O_2 + catalase \rightarrow H_2O \text{ and } O_2$$

Reactive nitrogen species (RNS: free radicals derived from nitrogen) are represented by nitric oxide (NO•). NO is synthesized by the enzyme nitric oxide synthase from L-arginine. NO• can combine with superoxide anion to form peroxynitrite, a powerful oxidant.

$$NO• + O_2•^- \rightarrow ONOO^- \text{ (peroxynitrite)}$$

When protonated (likely at physiological pH), peroxynitrite spontaneously decomposes to reactive nitric dioxide and hydroxyl radicals:

$$ONOO^- + H^+ \rightarrow •NO_2 + OH•$$

Superoxide dismutase (SOD) can also enhance the peroxynitrite-mediated nitration of tyrosine residues on critical proteins, presumably via species similar to the nitronium cation (NO_2^+):

$$ONOO^- \text{ plus } SOD \rightarrow NO_2^+ \rightarrow \text{ Nitration of tyrosine}$$

WHAT IS INFLAMMATION?

Inflammation in Latin is referred to as *inflammare,* which means "setting on fire." Inflammation is a complex biological response initiated by the immune system. It removes infective agents such as bacteria and viruses, and helps to repair tissue damage caused by ionizing radiation, toxic chemicals, and/or traumatic injuries to the body. Immune cells in the peripheral blood, such as neutrophils and macrophages, participate in inflammatory reactions. In the brain, microglia are considered to be the inflammatory cells.

Primary features of inflammation at the affected site include redness, swelling, and warmth when touched, in addition to varying degrees of pain. These characteristics of inflammation were first recognized by the renowned Roman medical scholar, Aulus Cornelius Celsus (circa 25 BCE to 50 CE).

The injured or infected cells release eicosanoids and cytokines. Growth factors and cytotoxic factors are also released. These cytokines and other chemicals recruit immune cells (white blood cells—leukocytes, macrophages, monocytes, lymphocytes, and plasma cells) to the site of infection to eliminate invading harmful organisms or to promote the healing of injured tissue (Martin and Leibovich 2005).

As the body removes the injurious infective microorganisms as well as initiates the healing process, the injured tissue is replaced by the regeneration of native parenchymal cells (original cell type), by filling of the injured site with fibroblastic tissue (scarring), or most commonly by a combination of both processes. During inflammation, toxic chemicals that may damage cells are also released.

TYPES OF INFLAMMATION

Inflammation is divided into two categories, acute and chronic. Acute inflammation occurs following cellular injury or infection with microorganisms. The period of acute inflammation is relatively short, lasting from a few minutes to a few days. The main features of acute inflammations are edema (accumulation of exudation of fluid and plasma in extracellular spaces) and the migration of leukocytes, primarily neutrophils, to the site of injury.

Chronic inflammation is a second form of inflammation. It occurs following persistent cellular injury or infection. The period of chronic inflammation is relatively long and can last as long as the injury or infection exists. The main features of chronic inflammation are the presence of lymphocytes and macrophages and the proliferation of blood vessels, fibrosis, and tissue necrosis.

Let's examine both types of inflammation in further detail below.

Acute Inflammation

Acute inflammation causes marked alterations in blood vessels, which allows plasma protein and leukocytes to leave the body's primary circulation pathways. Subsequently, the leukocytes migrate to the site of injury by a process called chemotaxis. Leukocytes engulf pathogenic organisms by phagocytosis and then kill them by generating bursts of reactive oxygen species (ROS) and other toxic substances. They can also engulf cellular debris and foreign antigens by a similar process and then degrade them with lysosomal proteolytic enzymes.

Leukocytes, however, may release excessive amounts of ROS, pro-inflammatory cytokines, prostaglandins, adhesion molecules, and complement proteins, and thus can damage normal tissue. An acute inflammatory reaction is tightly regulated and turned off soon after the injured sites are healed or the invading microbes removed.

Acute inflammation is an essential process for the removal of pathogens (harmful organisms) and cellular debris from the damaged site, thus allowing healing to occur. However, it is effective only when the injurious stimuli or tissue damage is relatively mild. If the tissue damage is extensive, or the levels of infective organisms are high, acute inflammatory reactions are not turned off. Consequently, the toxic products of these reactions can enhance the rate of damage, which may cause organ failure and eventually even death.

Chronic Inflammation

Persistent low-grade cellular injury or exposure to exogenous agents such as particulate silica or infection can initiate chronic inflammation. Chronic inflammation is often associated with most human neurodegenerative conditions and diseases.

In contrast to acute inflammation, which is characterized by vascular changes, edema, and primarily neutrophil infiltration, chronic inflammation is characterized by the presence of mononuclear cells, which include macrophages, lymphocytes, and plasma cells. In the brain, microglia cells become activated and migrate to the site of injury. During chronic inflammation the presence of angiogenesis and fibrosis can be observed at the site of injury.

Although the acute inflammatory responses may produce pro-inflammatory cytokines, reactive oxygen species (ROS), prostaglandins, adhesion molecules, and complements, the chronic inflammatory processes more typically do so. Therefore, they are more relevant to neuro-degenerative diseases when compared to acute inflammatory reactions. As we have learned, the release of these agents is tightly regulated and is mitigated when the invading pathogenic (harmful) organisms are killed or the injured tissues are healed. In chronic inflammation, on the other hand, the inflammatory response to chronic cellular injury or chronic infection is not turned off.

PRODUCTS OF INFLAMMATORY REACTIONS

As we know, during inflammation, several highly reactive agents are released. They include cytokines, complement proteins, arachidonic acid (AA) metabolites, ROS, and endothelial/leukocyte adhesion molecules. They are briefly described below.

Cytokines

Cytokines are proteins released during both acute and chronic inflammation. They are produced by many cell types primarily by activated lymphocytes and macrophages, but also by endothelium, epithelium, and connective tissue cells. In the brain, they are produced primarily by microglia cells and some by neurons. Pro-inflammatory cytokines include interleukin-6 (IL-6), IL-17, IL-18, IL-23, and tumor necrosis factor-alpha (TNF-alpha) that are toxic to the cells. Anti-inflammatory cytokines include IL-1, IL-4, IL-10, IL-11, and IL-13, which help in the repair at the site of injury.

If the tissue damage is severe, the pro-inflammatory cytokines may overcome the repair function of the anti-inflammatory cytokines, and participate in the progression of damage. Some pro-inflammatory cytokines such as IL-6 can also act as a neurotrophic factor. In this it functions as a pro-inflammatory cytokine during the acute phase of injury, and as a neurotrophic factor between the sub-acute and chronic phase of injury.

Cytokines play an important role in modulating the function of many other cell types. They are multifunctional, and individual cytokines may have both positive and negative regulatory actions. Cytokines mediate their action by binding to specific receptors on target cells. These receptors are regulated by exogenous and endogenous signals. Cytokines that regulate lymphocyte activation, growth, and differentiation include interleukin-2 (IL-2) and IL-4 (favors growth), as well as IL-10 and transforming growth factor-beta (TGF-beta) that are negative regulators of immune responses.

Cytokines involved with natural immunity include tumor necrosis factor-alpha (TNF-alpha), IL-1Beta, type I interferon (IFN-alpha and IFN-beta), and IL-6. Cytokines that activate inflammatory cells such as macrophages include IFN-gamma, TNF-alpha, TNF-beta, IL-5, IL-10, and IL-12. Cytokines that stimulate hematopoiesis (growth and differentiation of immature leukocytes) include IL-3, IL-7, c-kit ligand, granulocyte-macrophage colony-stimulating factor (GM-CSF), macrophage colony-stimulating factor (M-CSF), granulocyte CSF, and stem cell factor.

Chemokines are also cytokines that stimulate leukocyte movement and direct them to the site of injury during inflammation. Many classical growth factors may also act as cytokines, and conversely, many cytokines exhibit activities of growth factors.

Complement Proteins

During inflammation, twenty complement proteins including their cleavage (degradation) products are released into the plasma, and when activated they can cause cell lysis (death). They can also exhibit proteolytic activity. They participate in both innate and adaptive immunity for protection against pathogenic organisms, however, they are considered major humoral components of the innate immune response (Rus, Cudrici, and Niculescu 2005). Complement proteins participate in killing pathogenic microorganisms by the antibodies through complex mechanisms. Complement proteins are numbered C1 through C9. All of them have complex mechanisms of action on cells. Some complement proteins are also neurotoxic.

Arachidonic Acid (AA) Metabolites

Arachidonic acid is a 20-carbon fatty acid that is derived from dietary sources or is formed from the essential fatty acid linoleic acid. During inflammation, AA metabolites, also called eicosanoids, are released. These eicosanoids have diverse biological actions, depending upon the cell type, and they are synthesized by two major classes of enzymes: Cyclooxygenase (COX) for the synthesis of prostaglandins and thromboxanes, and lipooxygenase for the synthesis of leukotrienes and lipoxins. There are two isoforms of cyclooxygenase: COX1 and COX2.

Endothelial/Leukocyte Adhesion Molecules

The immunoglobulin family molecules include two endothelial adhesion molecules: intracellular adhesion molecule-1 (ICAM-1) and vascular adhesion molecule-1 (VCAM-1). These adhesion molecules bind with leukocyte receptor integrins. They are induced by IL-1 and TNF-alpha. Both ICAM-1 and VCAM-1 are released during inflammatory reactions and have diverse mechanisms of action on cells.

Leukocytes

Leukocytes include the phagocytes (primarily macrophages and neutrophils), and dendritic cells, mast cells, eosinophils, basophils, and natural killer cells. These cells identify and kill harmful microorganisms by phagocytosis. Phagocytosis is an important feature of cellular innate immunity. Neutrophils and macrophages are the most active in phagocytosis following infection with pathogenic microorganisms. These cells engulf pathogens that are trapped in an intracellular vesicle called phagosomes, which fuse with lysosomes to form phagolysosomes. The harmful organisms are killed by proteolytic enzymes (enzymes that can digest) of the lysosomes aided by burst of ROS released by the phagocytes. Natural killer cells can kill tumor cells or cells infected with viruses.

WHAT IS THE IMMUNE SYSTEM?

The immune system is a network of cells, tissues, and organs that works together in a highly coordinated manner to defend the body against foreign invading pathogenic organisms or antigenic molecules or particles. It plays an important role in defense against invading pathogenic (harmful) organisms, therefore, it's essential for survival. Under certain conditions, the immune system can produce toxic chemicals that play an important role in the initiation and progression of chronic neurodegenerative diseases as well as causing autoimmune diseases.

The immune system is highly complex and tightly regulated. On one hand, it defends the body against foreign invading pathogenic microorganisms and antigenic molecules or particles. On the other hand, it has the ability to produce toxic chemicals such as reactive oxygen species (ROS), pro-inflammatory cytokines, complement proteins, adhesion molecules, and prostaglandins, all of which are toxic to the tissues. These toxic chemicals may increase the risk of chronic conditions, including neurodegenerative conditions. Furthermore, the presence of endogenous antigens can initiate an immune response that damages body's own tissue such as is seen in rheumatoid arthritis.

Once the immune system has been exposed to an antigen and successfully removes it, it stores the recognition factor of this antigen in its memory. Thus, during the lifetime of an individual, the immune system stores recognition factors of millions of different antigens and thus protects the body from these antigens all the time. This process of exposure to an antigen and successfully removing it is generally referred to as acquired immunity, which is the basis of vaccination.

The organs of the immune system are located throughout the body. They are lymphoid organs than contain lymphocytes and bone marrow that contain all blood cells, including lymphocytes. Thymus-derived lymphocytes are referred to as T-lymphocytes (T-cells). In the blood, T-cell represents about 60–70 percent of peripheral lymphocytes. Lymphocytes derived from bone marrow are referred to as B-lymphocytes (B-cells). They constitute about 10–20 percent of peripheral lymphocytes in the blood. B-cells mature to plasma cells that secrete specific antibodies in response to a particular antigen.

Macrophages are derived from monocytes of bone marrow, and are a part of the mononuclear phagocyte system. They exhibit phagocytic activity, which is essential for removing harmful organisms from the body. A specialized form of cells with numerous fine dendritic cytoplasmic processes, called dendritic cells, does not exhibit phagocytic activity. They play an important role in presenting antigen to T-cells. Natural killer (NK) cells represent about 10–15 percent of the peripheral blood lymphocytes and lack T-cell receptors. They can kill tumor cells.

The major components of the immune system are innate immunity and adaptive immunity. The innate immune defenses are non-specific, but it is the dominant system of host defense (Litman, Cannon, and Dishaw 2005). The innate immune response is activated when microorganisms are identified by pattern of recognition receptors or when damaged cells send signals to immune system for a defensive response (Medzhitov 2007; Matzinger 2002). The innate immune responses do not confer long-lasting immunity against pathogenic organisms. The innate immune system responds to infection by inducing inflammation, releasing complement proteins, and recruiting leukocytes.

INNATE IMMUNITY

The components of innate immunity include inflammation, complement proteins, and leukocytes, all of which we have detailed earlier in this chapter. Innate immunity can activate adaptive immunity.

ADAPTIVE IMMUNITY

The adaptive response to an antigen is strong and is responsible for storing and re-calling immunologic memory for recognizing and eliminating a specific antigen all the time. The lymphocytes (T-cells and B-cells) are responsible for the adaptive immune response. Both T-cells and B-cells carry receptors that recognize specific targets. T-cells can recognize only membrane bound antigens. The cell surface major histocompatibility complex (MHC) molecules binds peptide fragments of foreign proteins for presentation to appropriate antigen-specific T-cells. There are two major subtypes of T-cells: the killer T-cells and the helper T-cells. The killer T-cells can recognize antigens bound to Class I MHC molecules, whereas the helper cells recognize antigens bound to Class II MHC molecules. A minor subtype of T-cells is $\gamma\delta$ T-cells that recognize intact antigens that are not bound to MHC receptors.

In contrast to the T-cells, the surface of B-cell has antibody molecule for a specific antigen. The antibody molecules recognize whole harmful organisms, and do not need any antigen presenting mechanism for their action. Each lineage of B-cell expresses a different antibody. A B-cell first identifies pathogens (harmful microorganism) when antibody on its surface binds to a specific foreign antigen. This antibody/antigen complex is engulfed by the B-cell where it is converted into peptides by proteolytic enzymes. The B-cells then display on their surface antigenic peptides and Class II MHC molecules that attract matching T-helper cells that release lymphokines and activate B-cells.

The activated B-cells proliferate and differentiate to plasma cells that secrete millions of copies of the antibody that recognize this antigen. These antibodies circulate in the blood and the lymph, and bind to pathogens expressing this particular antigen. These antibody/antigen bound pathogens are destroyed by complement protein activation or by phagocytes. Antibodies can also neutralize bacterial toxins by directly binding to them, and kill bacteria or viruses by interfering with their receptors that are used to infect cells.

CONCLUDING REMARKS

Free radicals are products of a biological process that occurs naturally as a result of the body's constant use of oxygen. For the last half a century, its significance as a contributory factor to the aging process has become more widely recognized, as has the understanding that it exists in part as an imbalance of our gene expression. Oxidative stress occurs when there is an excessive production of free radicals in the body; these may be derived from oxygen or from nitrogen. An excessive production of free radicals may pave the way for disease, given that an overabundance of toxic free radicals are capable of damaging the body's cells and tissues unless they can be neutralized by the body's defensive systems.

These defensive systems include the processes of antioxidant defense system, anti-inflammation products of inflammation, and the immune system itself. Antioxidants destroy free radicals. When one is injured or has an infection, the immune system immediately initiates actions to set a healing cascade in place. When this happens, white blood cells and anti-inflammatory compounds are called to the site of infection or injury to repair the damage. Once these agents have completed their work and the healing process is complete, the healing agents recede. However, if the immune system is compromised, or the injury overwhelms the imuune system, the cellular damage may persist, and a state of chronic inflammation may ensue.

The initiation and progression of most chronic neurodegenerative diseases are characterized by increased oxidative stress, chronic inflammation, and glutamate release. If these biological events can be adequately controlled and managed, one reduces the risk of developing the debilitating neurological conditions that are the subjects of this book.

3 The Antioxidant Defense System

This chapter presents a broad overview of antioxidants and as such, details many of their qualities and characteristics. This discussion is important for a more enhanced understanding of these valuable substances and will be a useful guide for those individuals seeking a greater inclusion of them through diet and/or supplementation. Specifically, the discussion in this chapter focuses on the history, functions, sources and forms, absorption, solubility, and availability of antioxidants. It also covers other practical matters such as how to most effectively store antioxidants in the home, whether or not they may be destroyed in cooking, and possible toxicity concerns.

It's vital to have this full complement of knowledge about antioxidants so that we may more completely understand the ensuing discussion in chapter 4. That discussion examines how, specifically, antioxidants help the body fight increased oxidative stress, inflammation, and glutamate release thereby helping to mitigate the effects of concussive injury, penetrating traumatic brain injury, and post-traumatic stress disorder.

A CLOSER LOOK AT ANTIOXIDANTS

Antioxidants are chemical micronutrients that donate an electron to a free radical and convert it into a harmless molecule. They are considered to be micronutrients. But what exactly is a micronutrient? In defining micronutrients it's important to distinguish them from macronutrients. Primarily, macronutrients include fats, carbohydrates, and proteins. Micronutrients, on the other hand, include antioxidant systems represented by dietary and endogenous antioxidant chemicals and antioxidant enzymes; polyphenolic compounds derived from fruits, vegetables, and plants; the mineral selenium; and B vitamins as well as vitamin D.

Although *all* micronutrients are essential for human survival and growth, antioxidants have enjoyed a special focus in this regard. They have been the subject of extensive laboratory research and clinical studies because of their potential importance in reducing oxidative stress and inflammation, which could decrease the risk of chronic disease.

Polyphenolic compounds derived from herbs also exhibit antioxidant and anti-inflammatory activities; however, they act in part by different mechanisms. Some of them reduce oxidative stress by activating the nuclear transcription factor Nrf2, which increases the levels of antioxidant enzymes by upregulating the antioxidant response element. Some dietary and endogenous antioxidants also activate Nrf2. Therefore, a combination of antioxidant chemicals and polyphenolic compounds may reduce oxidative stress and inflammation optimally.

The antioxidant defense system in humans can be divided into four groups, which we will look at next.

Group 1 Antioxidants

These antioxidants are not made in the body but are consumed primarily through the diet. They include vitamin A, carotenoids, vitamin C, vitamin E, and selenium. They scavenge free radicals directly.

Group 2 Antioxidants

Group 2 antioxidants are made in the body and are also consumed through the diet (primarily through meat and eggs), or in the form of supplements. They include glutathione, coenzyme Q10, reduced nicotinamide adenine dinucleotide (NADH), NAC, α-lipoic acid, and L-carnitine.

Group 3 Antioxidants

Group 3 antioxidants include antioxidants derived from fruit, vegetables, and plants. They also include polyphenolic compounds such as curcumin and resveratrol, which can be taken through the diet. However, dietary sources of these polyphenolic compounds may not provide sufficient amounts needed for the prevention of chronic neurological conditions. Thus supplementation may be necessary for optimal biological activity in the body. Both curcumin and resveratrol activate a nuclear transcriptional factor, Nrf2, which increases the levels of antioxidant enzymes through the antioxidant response element.

Group 4 Antioxidants

Another form of antioxidants are antioxidant enzymes that are made in the body. They include superoxide dismutase (SOD), catalase, and glutathione peroxidase. Superoxide dismutase requires manganese (Mn) or copper (Cu)-zinc SOD for its biological activity. Mn-SOD is present in the mitochondria, whereas Cu-Zn SOD is present in the cytoplasm. Both can destroy free radicals and hydrogen peroxide. Catalase requires iron (Fe) for its biological activity. It too, destroys hydrogen peroxide in the cell. Glutathione peroxidase requires selenium for its biological activity.

THE ROLE OF ANTIOXIDANTS

Antioxidants have many valuable roles to play in safeguarding human health. Given that they're so successful in neutralizing free radicals, many people believe that this is their only function. However, in view of recent advances in antioxidant research, this belief has been proven to be incorrect. The actions of antioxidants on cells and tissues are varied and complex. Antioxidants and polyphenolic compounds work to:

1. Scavenge free radicals
2. Decrease markers of pro-inflammatory cytokines
3. Alter gene expression profiles
4. Alter protein kinase activity
5. Prevent the release and toxicity of excessive amounts of glutamate
6. Act as co-factors for several biological reactions
7. Induce cell differentiation and apoptosis in cancer cells
8. Induce cell differentiation in normal cells, but not apoptosis
9. Increase immune function
10. Activate nuclear transcriptional factor Nrf2 that is essential for increasing the levels of antioxidant enzymes and phase-2-detoxyfying enzymes

HISTORY OF ANTIOXIDANTS

Vitamin A

Night blindness existed for centuries before the discovery of vitamin A. As early as 1500 BCE, Egyptians knew how to cure night blindness. Roman soldiers suffering from this condition traveled to Egypt where they received liver extract as treatment. (Today it is well established that liver is the richest source of vitamin A.) Treating night blindness with liver extract was not employed outside of Egypt for centuries, perhaps because medical establishments in other countries during that time period did not deem it to be an acceptable treatment protocol.

In 1912, Dr. Elmer McCollum of the University of Wisconsin discovered vitamin A in butter, at which time it was named "fat-soluble A." The structure of vitamin A was determined in 1930, and it was synthesized in the laboratory in 1947.

It should be underscored that the medical establishment of that very early period, by denying the validity of vitamin A to cure night blindness, no doubt delayed the cure for blindness for centuries.

The Vitamin B Family

All of the B vitamins were discovered between 1912 and 1934. In the year 1912, the Polish biochemist Dr. Casimur Funk isolated their active substances from the rice husks of unpolished rice; these active substances prevented the disease beriberi. This disease affects many parts of the body including muscle tissue, the heart, the nervous system, and the digestive tract. Dr. Funk named the substances he discovered vitamines, because he thought they were "amines" derived from ammonia. In 1920, the *e* was dropped when it became known that not all vitamins are "amines." Today there are many different vitamins in the vitamin B family.

Vitamin C

A vitamin C deficiency causes scurvy, the symptoms of which were known to Egyptians as early as 1500 BCE. In the fifth century Hippocrates described these symptoms. They include bleeding gums, hemorrhaging, and death. Native Americans had a cure for scurvy, which involved drinking an extract made from the bark and needles of the pine tree, prepared like a tea. This remedy, however, remained limited to their own population for hundreds of years. Today we know that pine bark and needles are rich in vitamin C.

During the sea voyages of European explorers between the twelfth and sixteenth centuries, the epidemic of scurvy among sailors forced some of them to land in Canada, where native Indians gave them the indigenous concoction, thereby curing their illness. In 1536, the French explorer Jacques Cartier brought this formulation to France, but the medical establishment rejected it as bogus because it had originated with the Native Americans, who they looked down upon. In 1593,

Sir Richard Hawkins began recommending that his sailors eat sour oranges and lemons to reduce the risk of disease. It would be almost another two hundred years before the British Navy began recommending that ships carry sufficient lime juice for all personnel aboard. In 1928, Albert Szent-Györgyi, a Hungarian scientist, isolated hexuronic acid from the adrenal gland. This substance was vitamin C, and in 1932 it was the first vitamin to be made in the laboratory.

It should be emphasized that the sixteenth-century medical community in France, by rejecting the use of vitamin C to treat scurvy, delayed the cure of this disease for centuries.

Carotenoids/Beta-Carotene

In 1919, carotenoid pigments were isolated from yellow plants, and in 1930 researchers found that some of the ingested carotene was converted to vitamin A. This substance is referred to as beta-carotene.

Vitamin D

Although the bone disease rickets may have existed in human populations for a long time, it wasn't until 1645 that Dr. Daniel Whistler described its symptoms. In 1922, Sir Edward Mellanby discovered vitamin D while working on a cure for rickets, which vitamin D proved to be. This vitamin was later found to require sunlight for its formation in skin cells. The chemical structure of vitamin D was determined by German scientist Dr. Adolf Windaus in 1930. Vitamin D_3 is the most active form of vitamin D. It was chemically characterized in 1936, and was initially thought to be a steroid effective in the treatment of rickets.

Vitamin E

In 1922, Dr. Herbert Evans of the University of California, Berkeley, observed that rats reared exclusively on whole milk grew normally but were not fertile. Fertility was restored when they were fed wheat germ.

However, it took another fourteen years before the active substance that was responsible for restoring fertility was isolated. When this was achieved, Dr. Evans named the substance tocopherol, from the Greek word meaning "to bear offspring," and then added *ol* to the end, signifying its chemical status as an alcohol.

FUNCTIONS OF
SPECIFIC ANTIOXIDANTS

Vitamin A

In addition to destroying free radicals, vitamin A plays an important role in maintaining vision and skin health; stimulating immune function; in bone metabolism; regulating gene activity, embryonic development, and reproduction; and inhibiting pre-cancerous and cancerous cell proliferation.

Alpha-lipoic Acid

Alpha-lipoic acid is a more potent antioxidant than vitamin C or vitamin E. It's soluble in both water and lipid and thus protects cellular membranes as well as water-soluble compounds. It regenerates tissue levels of vitamin C and vitamin E and markedly elevates glutathione level in the cells. Alpha-lipoic acid acts as a co-factor for multi-enzyme dehydrogenase complexes.

Vitamin C

Vitamin C acts as an antioxidant and participates as a cofactor for the activities of some enzymes, which is essential for the formation of many vital compounds in our body. Vitamin C helps in the formation of collagen, and it also takes part in the formation of interferon, a naturally occurring anti-viral agent. It regenerates oxidized vitamin E to a reduced form, which acts as an antioxidant.

Carotenoids

Beta-carotene is a precursor of vitamin A. Carotenes are known to protect against ultraviolet-light-induced damage. Beta-carotene increases the expression of the connexin gene, which codes for a gap junction protein that holds two normal cells together. (Vitamin A can't produce such an effect.) In addition, when compared to vitamins A and E, beta-carotene is a more effective destroyer of free radicals in an internal body environment that is marked by high oxygen pressure in the tissues.

Coenzyme Q10

Coenzyme Q10 is a weak antioxidant, but it recycles vitamin E. Coenzyme Q10 is essential in generating energy by the mitochondria.

Vitamin D₃

Vitamin D_3 is essential for bone formation, and regulates calcium and phosphorus levels in the blood. Vitamin D_3 also inhibits parathyroid hormone secretion from the parathyroid glands. It stimulates immune function by promoting phagocytosis and also exhibits anti-tumor activity.

Vitamin E

Vitamin E acts as an antioxidant and regulates gene expression. It also translocates certain proteins from one cellular compartment to another. Additionally, it helps to maintain skin texture, reduces scarring, and acts as an anticoagulant. Vitamin E reduces inflammation and stimulates immune function. Its derivative, vitamin E succinate, exhibits potent anticancer activities.

Glutathione

Glutathione is one of the most important antioxidants in that it protects cellular components inside the cells. It is needed for detoxi-fication, either of certain exogenous toxins or those generated as by-products of normal metabolism. Glutathione also acts as a substrate for several enzymes. It reduces inflammation.

Melatonin

Melatonin is important in regulating circadian rhythms through its receptor. It also acts as an antioxidant and reduces inflammation. Unlike other antioxidants, the oxidation of melatonin is irreversible, and thus cannot be regenerated by other antioxidants. Melatonin also stimulates immune function.

N-acetylcysteine (NAC)

N-acetylcysteine increases the glutathione levels within the cells. This function is important because orally administered glutathione is totally destroyed in the small intestine. At high doses, n-acetylcysteine binds with metals and removes them from the body.

Nicotinamide (Vitamin B₃)

Treatment with nicotinamide restored memory deficits in Alzheimer's disease transgenic mice (Green et al. 2008), attenuated glutamate-induced toxicity, and preserved cellular levels of NAD+ to support the activity of SIRT-1 (Liu, Pitta, and Mattson 2008). Treatment with nicotinamide reduced oxidative-stress-induced mitochondrial dysfunction and increased the survival of neurons in culture. The reduced form of NAD (NADH) acts as an antioxidant, and is essential for generating energy by the mitochondria.

Polyphenolic Compounds

Polyphenolic compounds exhibit antioxidant activity and reduce inflammation. They also regulate the expression of certain genes. Some polyphenolic compounds such as resveratrol and curcumin also increase the levels of antioxidant enzymes by activating a nuclear transcriptional factor, Nrf2.

SOURCES AND FORMS OF ANTIOXIDANTS

Vitamin A

Liver from beef, pork, chicken, turkey, and fish is the richest source of vitamin A (6.5 milligrams per 100 grams of liver). Other rich sources are carrot (0.8 milligrams per 100 grams), broccoli (0.8 milligrams per 100 grams), sweet potato (0.7 milligrams per 100 grams), kale (0.7 milligrams per 100 grams), butter (0.7 milligrams per 100 grams), spinach (0.5 milligrams per 100 grams), and pumpkin (0.4 milligrams per 100 grams). Minor sources include cantaloupe melon, egg, apricot, papaya, and mango (40 to 170 micrograms per 100 grams). Yellow and red fruits and vegetables are very rich sources of beta-carotene. One molecule of beta-carotene is converted to two molecules of retinol in the intestinal tract.

Vitamin A exists as retinyl palmitate or retinyl acetate that's converted into the retinol form in the body. Vitamin A exists as a retinoic acid in the cells. It has been determined that 1 IU (international unit) equals 0.3 micrograms of retinol, or 0.6 micrograms of beta-carotene. The activity of vitamin A is also expressed as retinol activity equivalent (RAE). One microgram of RAE corresponds to 1 microgram of retinol and 2 micrograms of beta-carotene in oil. Vitamin A, beta-carotene, and the synthetic retinoids are also available commercially.

Vitamin C

The richest source of vitamin C is fruits and vegetables, which include rose hip (2,000 milligrams per 100 grams of rose hip), red pepper (2,000 milligrams per 100 grams of red pepper), parsley (2,000 milligrams per 100 grams of parsley), guava (2,000 milligrams per 100 grams of guava), kiwi fruit (2,000 milligrams per 100 grams of kiwi fruit), broccoli (2,000 milligrams per 100 grams of broccoli), lychee (2,000 milligrams per 100 grams of lychee), papaya (2,000 milligrams per 100 grams of papaya), and strawberry (2,000 milligrams per 100 grams of strawberry). Other sources of vitamin C include orange, lemon, melon, garlic, cauliflower, grapefruit, raspberry, tangerine, passion fruit, spinach, and lime. These foods contain about 30 to 50 milligrams per 100 grams of fruits and vegetables. Vitamin C is sold commercially as L-ascorbic acid, calcium ascorbate, sodium ascorbate, and potassium ascorbate.

Carotenoids
The richest sources of carotenoids are sweet potato, carrot, spinach, mango, cantaloupe, apricot, kale, broccoli, parsley, cilantro, pumpkin, winter squash, and fresh thyme. There are two main forms of carotenoids found in nature: alpha-carotene and beta-carotene. Beta-carotene is one of the more than 600 carotenoids found in fruits, vegetables, and plants, and represents the more common form of carotenoids. Other carotenes include lutein and lycopene.

Coenzyme Q10
In 1957, Dr. Fredrick Crane isolated coenzyme Q10. In 1958, Dr. Wolf, working under Dr. Karl Folkers, determined the structure of coenzyme Q10.

Vitamin E
The richest sources of vitamin E include wheat germ oil (215 milligrams per 100 grams of oil), sunflower oil (56 milligrams per 100 grams of oil), olive oil (12 milligrams per 100 grams of oil), almond oil (39 milligrams per 100 grams of oil), hazelnut oil (26 milligrams per 100 grams of oil), walnut oil (20 milligrams per 100 grams of oil), and peanut oil (17 milligrams per 100 grams of oil). The sources for small amounts of vitamin E (0.1 to 2 milligrams per 100 grams) include kiwi fruit, fish, leafy vegetables, and whole grains. In the United States, fortified breakfast cereal is an important source of vitamin E. At present, the natural form of vitamin E is primarily extracted from vegetable oil, particularly soybean oil.

Vitamin E exists in eight different forms: four tocopherols (alpha-, beta-, gamma-, and delta-tocopherol), and four tocotrienols (alpha-, beta-, gamma-, and delta-tocotrienol). Alpha-tocopherol has the most biological activity. Vitamin E exists in the natural form commonly indicated as "d" whereas the synthetic form is referred to as "dl." The stable esterified form of vitamin E is available as alpha-tocopheryl acetate, alpha-tocopheryl succinate, and alpha-tocopheryl nicotinate. The activity of vitamin E is generally expressed in international units (IU). It is determined that 1 IU equals 0.66 milligrams of d-alpha-tocopherol, and 1 IU of racemic mixture (dl-form) equals 0.45 milligrams of d-tocopherol.

Glutathione

Glutathione is synthesized from three amino acids: L-cysteine, L-glutamic acid, and L-glycine, and is present in all cells of the body, however, its highest concentration is found in the liver. Glutathione exists in the cells in a reduced or oxidized form. In healthy cells, more than 90 percent of glutathione is present in the reduced form. The oxidized form of glutathione can be converted to the reduced form by the enzyme glutathione reductase. The reduced form of glutathione acts as an antioxidant.

L-carnitine

L-carnitine was originally found to be a growth factor for mealworms. It is synthesized, primarily in the liver and kidney from the amino acids lysine and methionine. Vitamin C is necessary for its synthesis. It exists as R-L-carnitine, a biologically active form, and as D-carnitine, a biologically inactive form.

Polyphenolic Compounds

Polyphenolic compounds are found in herbs, fruits, vegetables, and plants. They include tannins, lignins, and flavonoids. The most widely studied polyphenolic compounds are flavonoids, which include resveratrol (in grape skin and seed), curcumin (in spices such as turmeric), ginseng extract, cinnamon extract, garlic extract, quercetin, epicatechin, and oligomeric proanthocyanidins. Major sources of flavonoids include all citrus fruit, berries, ginkgo biloba, onion, parsley, tea, red wine, and dark chocolate. Over five thousand naturally occurring flavonoids have been characterized from various plants.

ABSORPTION OF ANTIOXIDANTS

Antioxidants are absorbed from the intestinal tract and then distributed to various organs of the body. The highest levels of vitamin A, C, and E are present in the liver, and the lowest levels of these antioxidants are in the brain. Regarding coenzyme Q10, the heart and the liver have the highest levels of it. Only about 10 percent of ingested water-soluble and fat-soluble antioxidants are absorbed from the intestinal tract. It has been argued by some that 90 percent of antioxidants are therefore wasted but this argument has no scientific merit.

During the process of digestion, many toxic substances including mutagens (agents that can alter genetic activity) and carcinogens (agents that can cause cancer) are formed. What's interesting to note is that the consumption of organic food makes little difference in the amount of toxins formed during the digestive process. Organic food may, however, be devoid of pesticides, although these pesticides represent only about 1 percent of naturally occurring toxins. Pesticides are not metabolized and are difficult to remove from the body.

The formation of toxins is more prevalent in meat eaters than in vegetarians. A portion of them are absorbed from the gut, and could increase the risk of chronic disease developing over a long period of time. The presence of excessive amounts of antioxidants markedly reduced the levels of toxins formed during digestion, and thereby reduced the risk of chronic disease development. Thus it is clear that unabsorbed antioxidants perform a very useful function in reducing the levels of mutagens and carcinogens formed during the digestion of food.

SOLUBILITY OF ANTIOXIDANTS AND POLYPHENOLIC COMPOUNDS

The lipid-soluble antioxidants include vitamin A, vitamin E, carotenoids, coenzyme Q10, and L-carnitine. Water-soluble antioxidants include vitamin C, glutathione, and alpha-lipoic acid. Polyphenolic compounds are generally fat-soluble. Fat-soluble vitamins and polyphenolic compounds should be taken with meals so that they are more readily absorbed.

AVAILABILITY OF ANTIOXIDANTS

Vitamin A
Vitamin A is commercially sold as retinyl palmitate, retinyl acetate, and retinoic acid and its analogues. Retinyl acetate or retinyl palmitate is converted to retinol in the intestine before absorption. Retinol is converted to retinoic acid in the cells. Retinoic acid performs all of the functions of vitamin A except for maintaining good vision. Retinol is stored in the liver as retinyl palmitate. Vitamin A exists as a protein-bound molecule. The level of retinol can be determined in the plasma.

Vitamin C
Vitamin C is commercially sold as ascorbic acid, sodium ascorbate, magnesium ascorbate, calcium ascorbate, and timed-release capsules containing ascorbic acid and vitamin C-ester. It is present in all cells. Ascorbic acid is converted to dehydroascorbic acid, which can be reduced to form vitamin C. It's interesting to note that dehydroascorbic acid can cross the blood-brain barrier, but vitamin C cannot. All mammals make vitamin C except guinea pigs. An adult goat makes

about thirteen grams of vitamin C every day. The plasma level of vitamin C may not reflect the tissue level of vitamin C, but in humans it's difficult to obtain tissues in order to determine vitamin C levels. Vitamin C can recycle oxidized vitamin E to the reduced form, which acts as an antioxidant.

Carotenoids

Beta-carotene is one of more than six hundred carotenoids found in fruits, vegetables, and plants. It is commercially available in natural or synthetic forms. The natural form of beta-carotene is more effective than the synthetic form. Preparations of natural carotenoids contain primarily beta-carotene; however, the other type of carotenoid is also present. A portion of ingested beta-carotene is converted to retinol (vitamin A) in the intestinal tract before absorption, and the remainder is distributed in the blood and tissues of the body. One molecule of beta-carotene forms two molecules of vitamin A. In humans, the conversion of beta-carotene to vitamin A doesn't occur if the body has sufficient amounts of vitamin A. Beta-carotene is primarily stored in the eyes and fatty tissues. Other carotenoids such as lycopene accumulate in the prostate more than in any other organ, whereas lutein accumulates in the eyes more than in any other organ.

Coenzyme Q10

About 95 percent of energy is generated from the use of coenzyme Q10 by the mitochondria. Therefore, organs such as the heart and liver that require high energy have the highest concentrations of coenzyme Q10. Other organelles inside the cells that contain coenzyme Q10 include endoplasmic reticulum, peroxisomes, lysosomes, and Golgi apparatus.

Vitamin E

Among vitamin E isomers, alpha-tocopherol is biologically more active than others. In recent years the research on tocotrienols has revealed some important biological functions. Vitamin E is commercially sold as d-or dl-tocopherol, alpha-tocopheryl acetate (vitamin E acetate), or alpha-tocopheryl succinate (vitamin E succinate). The esterified form of vitamin E (vitamin E acetate and vitamin E succinate) are more stable than alpha-tocopherol. Vitamin E acetate has been widely used in basic research and clinical studies.

It's been presumed that vitamin E acetate or vitamin E succinate is converted to alpha-tocopherol in the intestinal tract before absorption. This assumption may be true for vitamin E succinate. If the body's stores of alpha-tocopherol are saturated, vitamin E succinate can be absorbed. Vitamin E succinate enters the cells more easily than alpha-tocopherol because of its greater solubility. As well, vitamin E succinate has some unique functions that cannot be produced by alpha-tocopherol.

Vitamin E succinate is now considered the most effective form of vitamin E, but it cannot act as an antioxidant until converted to alpha-tocopherol. Alpha-tocopherol is located primarily in the membranous structures of the cells. The level of vitamin E can be determined in the plasma.

Glutathione and Alpha-lipoic Acid

Glutathione is the most important antioxidant within the cells and it is present in all cells. Although it's sold commercially for oral consumption, it's totally destroyed in the intestine. Therefore, oral administration of glutathione doesn't increase the cellular level of glutathione, however, n-acetylcysteine (NAC) does. In the body, n-acetyl is removed from NAC by the enzyme esterase, and then cysteine is used to synthesize glutathione.

Alpha-lipoic acid also increases the cellular levels of glutathione by a mechanism that differs from the mechanism of NAC.

L-carnitine

L-carnitine is made in the body, but we can also obtain it from the diet. The highest concentration of L-carnitine is found in red meat (95 milligrams per 3.0 ounces of meat). In contrast, the chicken breast has only 3.9 milligrams per 3.5 ounces. L-carnitine is present in all of the cells of our body.

Melatonin

Melatonin is a naturally occurring hormone produced primarily by the pineal gland in the brain. It is also produced by the retina, the lens, and the gastrointestinal tract. Melatonin is synthesized from the amino acid tryptophan. It is also present in various plants such as rice. It is readily absorbed from the intestinal tract; however, 50 percent of it is removed from the plasma in thirty-five to fifty minutes. It has several biological functions including antioxidant and anti-inflammatory activities. Melatonin is necessary for the proper regulation of sleep cycles.

Nicotinamide (Vitamin B3) and Nicotinamide Adenine Dinucleotide Dehydrogenase (NADH)

Treatment with nicotinamide, a precursor of nicotinamide adenine dinucleotide (NAD^+), reduced oxidative stress-induced mitochondrial dysfunction and increased the survival of neurons in culture. Nicotinamide also attenuated glutamate-induced toxicity. Histone deacetylase inhibitors increase histone acetylation and enhance memory and neuronal plasticity. Nicotinamide (vitamin B3), an inhibitor of histone deacetylase activity, restored memory deficits in Alzheimer's transgenic mice. Thus, the addition of nicotinamide to a preparation of micronutrients may be necessary in order to reduce the risk of developing memory loss and to increase the survival of neurons in neurodegenerative diseases.

Nicotinamide adenine dinucleotide (NAD^+) and NADH (the reduced form of NAD) are present in all of the cells of our body.

NAD^+ is an oxidizing agent, therefore, it can act as a pro-oxidant, whereas NADH can act as an antioxidant. NAD^+ accepts electrons from other molecules and is reduced to form NADH. NADH can recycle oxidized vitamin E to the reduced form, which can act as an antioxidant. NADH is essential for mitochondria to generate energy.

Polyphenolic Compounds

Flavonoids (polyphenolic compounds) are poorly absorbed by the intestinal tract in humans. All of them possess varying degrees of antioxidants and anti-inflammatory activities.

HOW TO STORE ANTIOXIDANTS

Vitamin A

Crystal forms of retinol, retinoic acid, retinyl acetate, and retinal palmitate can be stored at 4°C for several months. A solution of retinoic acid is stable at 4°C, stored away from light, for several weeks.

Vitamin C

Vitamin C should not be stored in solution form because it is easily destroyed within a few days. The crystal or tablet forms of vitamin C can be kept at room temperature, away from light, for a few years.

Carotenoids

Most commercially sold carotenoids in solid form can be stored at room temperature away from light for a few years. Beta-carotene in solution, however, degrades within a few days, even when stored in a colder environment away from light.

Coenzyme Q10 and NADH

These antioxidants in solid forms are stable when stored at room temperature, away from light, for few years. The solutions of these antioxidants are stable when stored at 4°C away from light for several months.

Vitamin E

Alpha-tocopherol is relatively unstable at room temperature in comparison to alpha-tocopheryl acetate and alpha-tocopheryl succinate. Alpha tocopherol can be stored at 4°C for several weeks, but alpha-tocopheryl acetate and alpha-tocopheryl succinate can be stored at room temperature for a few years. A solution of alpha-tocopheryl succinate is stable for several months at 4°C if kept away from the light.

Glutathione, N-acetylcysteine, and Alpha-Lipoic Acid

Solid forms of glutathione, n-acetylcysteine, and alpha-lipoic acid are stable at room temperature away from light, for a few years. The solutions of these antioxidants are stable when stored at 4°C, away from light, for several months.

Melatonin

The powdered form of melatonin is stable at 4°C for a year or more.

Polyphenolic Compounds

Polyphenolic compounds are very stable at room temperature, away from light, for a few years.

CAN ANTIOXIDANTS BE DESTROYED DURING COOKING?

Vitamin A

Routine cooking does not destroy vitamin A, but slow heating for a long period of time may reduce its potency. Canning and prolonged cold storage may also diminish its activity. The vitamin A content of fortified milk powder declines substantially after two years.

Carotenoids

Most carotenes, especially lutein and lycopene, are not destroyed during cooking. In fact, their bioavailability improves when they're derived from a cooked or extracted preparation, for example, lycopene from tomato sauce.

Coenzyme Q10 and NADH

Coenzyme Q10 and NADH can be partially degraded during cooking.

Vitamin E

Food processing, frying, and freezing destroy vitamin E. The vitamin E content of fortified milk powder is unaffected over a two-year period.

Glutathione, N-acetylcysteine, and Alpha-lipoic Acid

Glutathione, n-acetylcysteine, and alpha-lipoic acid can be partially destroyed during cooking.

Polyphenolic Compounds

Polylphenolic compounds are not destroyed during cooking.

TOXICITY OF MICRONUTRIENTS

Some micronutrients may produce harmful effects, but only when consumed at relatively high doses over a long period of time. For example, vitamin A at doses of 10,000 IU or more per day can cause birth defects in pregnant women, and beta-carotene at doses of 50 milligrams or more can produce bronzing of the skin that is reversible on discontinuation. Vitamin C as ascorbic acid at high doses (10 grams or more per day) can cause diarrhea in some individuals. Vitamin E at high doses (2,000 IU or more per day) can induce clotting defects after long-term consumption. Vitamin B6 at high doses (50 milligrams or more per day) may produce peripheral neuropathy, and selenium at doses 400 micrograms or more per day can cause skin and liver toxicity after long-term consumption. Coenzyme Q10 has no known toxicity, and recommended daily doses are 30–400 milligrams. N-acetylcysteine (NAC) doses of 250–1500 milligrams and alpha-lipoic acid doses of 600 milligrams are used in humans without toxicity.

CONCLUDING REMARKS

Early in the mists of time, when life on the planet consisted primarily of small anaerobic organisms, oxygen as we know it today did not yet exist. However, these organisms eventually acquired the ability to break water down into its constituent parts of hydrogen and oxygen. Because the newly generated oxygen was toxic to these organisms they had to adapt to it in order to survive. They did this by developing defensive systems that would protect them from oxidative damage. As these organisms evolved into humans, defensive antioxidant shields evolved with them.

When the body processes oxygen, free radicals are created. Infection and metabolism are two additional processes that generate free radicals in the body. As well, certain trace minerals (iron, copper, and manganese, in combination with molecules like vitamin C and uric acid) can also form free radicals. These free radicals may overwhelm the body's antioxidant system, thus underscoring the need to ensure the presence of large amounts of antioxidants in the body at all times.

There are many different types of antioxidants: those that are made in the body and those that are derived from outside sources via either diet or dietary supplement. In terms of dietary antioxidants and guidance regarding their consumption, it's useful to refer to the

Daily Recommended Intake, which is an index established for each micronutrient. The DRI is found in the appendix of this book. (The DRI replaces the former index known as the Recommended Dietary Allowance). However, it must be noted that although these recommended doses allow for normal growth and development, they're not optimal for reducing increased oxidative stress and inflammation.

In the next chapter we will examine the role that antioxidants play in reducing chronic inflammation and increased oxidative stress by looking at how they are currently perceived by the medical community and what that means for the future exploration of treating concussive injury, penetrating traumatic brain injury, and post-traumatic stress disorder.

4 The Role of Antioxidants in Reducing Oxidative Damage

Despite the fact that antioxidants are so essential for our growth and survival, they remain misunderstood and misused by most of the public as well as by a majority of health care professionals. The reasons for this include inaccurate claims by many in the nutrition industry, inconsistent human data (stemming from epidemiologic studies), and the results of poorly designed clinical studies in which one or sometimes two antioxidants in populations at high risk for developing chronic diseases were administered.

Despite basic scientific evidence attesting to the importance of multiple antioxidants in disease prevention and improvement in the management of chronic diseases, when antioxidants are used in combination with standard therapy the medical establishment is not convinced of their value. This is not the first time that the medical establishment has resisted the application of these novel agents in the treatment of disease. The history of the discovery of vitamin A and vitamin C illustrates how the cure for night blindness and scurvy was delayed for centuries because of resistance by the medical establishment.

In this chapter, we will examine optimal types and doses of

antioxidants that should be utilized in the prevention of disease. We will examine how best to reduce oxidative stress, chronic inflammation, and glutamate release in the body. We will also discuss prevailing norms and attitudes about antioxidant use, which has resulted in flawed human studies as regards the potentially curative effects of these important substances.

MISUSE OF ANTIOXIDANTS IN CLINICAL STUDIES FOR PREVENTION OF CHRONIC DISEASES

For growth and survival, humans need dietary antioxidants (vitamins A, C, E, and carotenoids, and the mineral selenium) as well as endogenous antioxidants made by the body. These endogenous antioxidants include antioxidant enzymes, glutathione, coenzyme Q10, R-alpha-lipoic acid, L-carnitine, and reduced nicotinamide adenine dinucleotide (NADH). The distribution of these antioxidants varies markedly from one organ to another, even within the same cell. Their sub-cellular distribution also differs markedly from one cellular compartment to another within the same cell.

The human body generates different types of inorganic and organic free radicals derived from oxygen and nitrogen in response to the utilization of oxygen. The exposure to various environmental stressors, such as ozone, dust particles, smoke, toxic fumes, toxic chemicals, and ionizing radiation (X-rays or gamma rays), also produces excessive amounts of free radicals. Free radical-induced damage is called oxidative damage; it also occurs during the normal aging process and during the initiation and progression of certain neurodegenerative conditions and diseases. Elevation of dietary and endogenous antioxidant chemicals as well as antioxidant enzymes is needed to reduce oxidative stress and inflammation optimally.

The affinities of antioxidants to specific types of free radicals differ and their efficacy in reducing oxidative damage may also differ. Some antioxidants also reduce the levels of chronic inflammation and reduce glutamate release and its toxicity.

These observations make it clear that supplementation with one or two dietary or endogenous antioxidants may not be useful in reducing the progression of damage in patients with acute or chronic neurodegenerative diseases. I propose that supplementation with a preparation of micronutrients containing dietary and endogenous antioxidants, B vitamins, vitamin D, selenium, certain phenolic compounds (curcumin and resveratrol), and omega-3 fatty acids may be essential for reducing the risk of developing as well as of slowing the progression of chronic neurodegenerative diseases. Unfortunately, nearly all previous clinical studies have utilized just one or two dietary antioxidants in populations that are at a high risk for developing certain chronic diseases, yielding inconsistent results.

Let's scrutinize what's involved in an optimally designed clinical study next.

OPTIMAL TYPES AND DOSES OF ANTIOXIDANTS

When designing a human clinical study, the *type* of antioxidant employed is key. For example, it's been reported that natural beta-carotene prevented the X-ray-induced transformation (cancer formation) of normal mouse fibroblasts in culture, whereas synthetic beta-carotene did not. An animal study showed that various organs accumulated the natural form of vitamin E (d-alpha-tocopherol) more than the synthetic form (dl-alpha-tocopherol). Furthermore, it has been reported that vitamin E in the form of d-alpha-tocopheryl succinate is more effective than other forms of vitamin E. Human studies with antioxidants have not taken these important issues into consideration; therefore, results pertaining to the efficacy of antioxidants have been contradictory.

The *doses* of antioxidants utilized are also very important in preventing disease and producing optimal health benefits. Low doses (those approximating DRI/RDA values) may be useful in reducing some oxidative damage and preventing deficiency, however, they may not be sufficient in reducing inflammation or optimizing immune function. The differences in changes in the expression of gene profiles between low and high doses of an antioxidant are very marked. In commercially sold multivitamin preparations, the dose amounts of antioxidants and other micronutrients vary markedly.

The *dose-schedule* of antioxidant micronutrients is also very critical in achieving the desired health benefits. Most people take micronutrient supplements once a day, which may not produce an optimal result. This is due to the fact that there is a high degree of fluctuation in the levels of antioxidants in the body because of a variation in the plasma half-lives of different micronutrients. In addition, as noted above, the expression of cell gene profiles differs markedly, depending on the level of antioxidants in the body. A once-a-day dose-schedule may compel the cells to constantly adjust their genetic activity due to variations in antioxidant levels in the body. Such a large fluctuation in genetic activity may not be desirable for optimal cell functioning. It's interesting to note that all previous human studies with antioxidants have utilized this once-a-day dose-schedule in spite of scientific evidence indicating that it is far from ideal.

In all human studies with antioxidants, the selection of the target population and the statistical analyses have been appropriate, but the selection of antioxidants, their doses, and dose-schedule have been designed without any real scientific rationale. This can be demonstrated by an examination of some widely publicized results of antioxidant studies as follows.

FLAWED ANTIOXIDANT STUDIES IN HUMANS

In a clinical study, the synthetic form of beta-carotene was administered orally once a day to males who were heavy tobacco smokers, in order to reduce the incidence of lung cancer. The results showed that the incidence of lung cancer in smokers who were treated with beta-carotene increased by about 17 percent (Albanes et al. 1995). Federal agencies and some nutrition scientists then promoted the idea that supplementation with beta-carotene may be harmful to one's health and recommended that consumers not take beta-carotene in any form or in any multivitamin preparation. These erroneous conclusions and recommendations were without any scientific merit for the following reasons.

It had been known before the start of this particular study that individual antioxidants such as beta-carotene can be oxidized in a high oxidative environment to become a pro-oxidant. Heavy tobacco smokers have a high internal oxidative environment. Therefore, when beta-carotene is administered to smokers, it is oxidized and acts as a pro-oxidant rather than as an antioxidant. Thus the expected outcome *would be* an increase in the incidence of cancer in tobacco smokers.

In contrast to the adverse effects of beta-carotene in heavy tobacco smokers, the same dose and type of beta-carotene did not increase the incidence of cancer among doctors and nurses who were nonsmokers during a five-year follow-up (Hennekens et al. 1996). Again, this result was also expected because populations of nonsmokers do not have a high internal oxidative environment.

Studies have also been done utilizing only vitamin E. Studies utilizing its natural and synthetic forms have produced inconsistent results in patients at high risk for the development of cardiovascular disease who also have an elevated internal oxidative environment. Some studies showed beneficial effects, whereas others showed no effect—or even adverse effects in some cases (Tornwall et al. 2004a; Tornwall et al. 2004b; Leppala et al. 2000; Yusuf et al. 2000).

The harmful effects of vitamin E alone on cardiovascular disease can be attributed to the same biological events as those observed with beta-carotene. At this time, cardiologists do not recommend vitamin E to their patients. There are no human data (intervention studies) to show that the same dose of vitamin E or beta-carotene, when present in an appropriately prepared multivitamin formula that includes dietary and endogenous antioxidants, produces adverse health effects among normal or high-risk populations.

Human studies featuring a single antioxidant have also produced inconsistent results in neurological diseases such as Parkinson's disease and Alzheimer's. In both studies, high doses of the synthetic form of vitamin E (800 IU per day in the case of Parkinson's, and 2,000 IU per day in the case of Alzheimer's) were used. No beneficial effects of vitamin E were observed in the study involving Parkinson's disease but some beneficial effects were observed in the study pertaining to early phase Alzheimer's disease (Sano et al. 1997). These studies were undertaken without a careful consideration of the biochemical factors involved in the disease processes or the antioxidant status of the patients involved.

It's been reported that a deficiency of the antioxidant glutathione is found in patients with Alzheimer's and Parkinson's disease. In addition, dysfunction of the mitochondria is consistently observed in the autopsied brains of patients with Parkinson's and Alzheimer's. Evidence of high oxidative damage and chronic inflammation has also been found in the brains of these patients. Therefore, the idea of supplementation with antioxidants to prevent or reduce the rate of progression of these diseases is an idea with merit. Supplementation with a multiple micronutrient preparation that contains appropriate doses of dietary and endogenous antioxidants, including glutathione-elevating agents as well as antioxidants that improve the function of the mitochondria to generate energy, would be beneficial in this context.

It's very unfortunate that the harmful results obtained with the use of primarily one antioxidant in high-risk populations are often extrapolated to all multiple antioxidant preparations and all populations. This erroneous extrapolation of data regarding the harmful effects of beta-carotene or vitamin E alone, for instance, is further propagated by the publication of meta-analysis of published data on the same vitamins with the same conclusion. A meta-analysis publication is often misinterpreted to be an original study. In my opinion, a meta-analysis should critically examine an experiment's design instead of just summarizing various study results.

Due to the fact that these studies are so poorly and inconsistently designed, their extrapolations have created a wide disconnect between the public and most health care professionals—especially physicians—regarding the health benefits of micronutrients. In an attempt to rectify this misunderstanding, in the subsequent chapters of this book I discuss the scientific basis for utilizing multiple micronutrients, including dietary and endogenous antioxidants in reducing the risk of developing neurodegenerative diseases. In addition, the role of these micronutrients in improving the efficacy of standard therapy for these diseases is also discussed.

THE REDUCTION OF OXIDATIVE STRESS, CHRONIC INFLAMMATION, AND GLUTAMATE RELEASE IN THE BODY

As we know, significant studies have suggested that increased oxidative stress, chronic inflammation, and the release of glutamate are involved in the progression of neurodegenerative conditions such as are discussed in this book. Therefore, reducing the levels of these harmful biological processes may prevent or otherwise slow the development of these neurodegenerative diseases, and in combination with standard therapy, may improve the management of them. This is where a formulation of the right combination of micronutrients becomes relevant.

How to Reduce Oxidative Stress

Oxidative stress occurs in the body when the antioxidant system fails to provide adequate protection against damage produced by free radicals (reactive oxygen species and reactive nitrogen species). Increased oxidative stress in the body can be most effectively reduced by upregulating the levels of antioxidant enzymes as well as by elevating the levels of dietary and endogenous antioxidant chemicals because they work, in part, by different mechanisms. For example, antioxidant enzymes reduce free radicals by catalysis (converting them into harmless molecules by a chemical reaction), whereas dietary and endogenous antioxidant chemicals reduce free radicals by directly scavenging them.

As mentioned previously, in response to reactive oxygen species (ROS), a nuclear transcriptional factor, Nrf2 (nuclear factor-erythroid 2-related factor 2), translocates from the cytoplasm to the nucleus where it binds with antioxidant response element (ARE), which increases the levels of antioxidant enzymes in order to reduce oxidative damage (Itoh et al. 1997; Hayes et al. 2000; Chan, Han, and Kan 2001). This normal response of activating Nrf2 becomes impaired in chronic neurodegenerative diseases. This is evidenced by the fact that in these diseases, increased oxidative stress continues to occur despite the presence of Nrf2. Therefore agents that activate Nrf2 by a ROS-independent mechanism must be identified. However, activation of Nrf2 may not be sufficient to optimally reduce oxidative stress. In response to increased oxidative stress, the levels of antioxidant chemicals in the body also decrease; therefore their levels must also be elevated for optimally reducing oxidative stress.

The levels of antioxidant chemicals cannot be elevated without supplementation.

Factors Regulating Response of Nrf2 and Its Action

Several studies exist to support the conclusion that antioxidant enzymes are elevated by Nrf2 activation, which depends upon ROS-dependent

(Niture et al. 2010) and independent mechanisms (Xi et al. 2012; Li et al. 2012; Bergstrom et al. 2011; Wruck et al. 2008; Hine and Mitchell 2012).

As part of this process, the levels of antioxidant enzymes are dependent upon the binding ability of Nrf2 with ARE in the nucleus (Suh et al. 2004).

Differential Response of Nrf2 to ROS
Generated During Acute and Chronic Oxidative Stress

In terms of ROS production, it appears that Nrf2 responds differently to *acute* oxidative stress than it does to *chronic* oxidative stress. For example, excessive amounts of ROS are generated during the acute oxidative stress observed in an individual undergoing strenuous exercise. In response to the increased ROS, as we know, Nrf2 translocates from the cytoplasm to the nucleus where it binds with ARE to upregulate antioxidant genes. Excessive amounts ROS are also present during chronic oxidative stress commonly found in older individuals and in individuals with neurological diseases such as Parkinson's disease, Alzheimer's disease, and post-traumatic stress disorder, suggesting that the Nrf2/ARE regulatory system has become unresponsive to ROS in these diseases.

Age-related decline in antioxidant enzymes in the liver of older rats compared to that in younger rats was due to reduction in the binding ability of Nrf2 with ARE. However, treatment with alpha-lipoic acid restored this defect, increased the levels of antioxidant enzymes, and restored the loss of glutathione from the liver of old rats (Suh et al. 2004). The exact reasons for the Nrf2/ARE regulatory system to become unresponsive to ROS during chronic oxidative stress are unknown; however, defects in the binding ability of Nrf2 with ARE may be part of the answer.

The levels of Nrf2 in the nucleus decreased in the hippocampal neurons of patients with Alzheimer's despite increased oxidative stress

(Ramsey et al. 2007). This suggests that the Nrf2/ARE pathway in Alzheimer's also becomes unresponsive to ROS stimulation, resulting in reduced translocation from the cytoplasm to the nucleus. It is also possible that the Nrf2 binding ability with ARE is impaired. It is not known whether the defect in the Nrf2 pathway occurs in the cytoplasm where Nrf2 forms a complex with Keap1 (an inhibitor of Nrf2) or at the level of the nucleus where it binds with ARE to enhance the expression of antioxidant genes—or at both levels.

Treatment with tert-butylhydroquinone, a known inducer of Nrf2, protected neurons against beta-amyloid-induced damage to the nerve cells in transgenic Alzheimer's mice. Insertion of the Nrf2 gene into the nerve cells protected them from the damaging effects of beta-amyloids (Kanninen et al. 2008).

No studies have been performed to evaluate the role of Nrf2 in concussive injury, penetrating TBI, or PTSD. However, the following groups of agents demonstrate that some antioxidant chemicals and polyphenolic compounds (curcumin and resveratrol) may have a dual function, given that they decrease oxidative stress by increasing antioxidant enzymes through activating the Nrf2/ARE pathway. As well, they scavenge free radicals directly. These agents are listed here.

1. Antioxidant chemicals scavenge free radicals. All dietary and endogenous antioxidant chemicals reduce varying levels of oxidative stress by directly scavenging free radicals.

2. Antioxidants and plant-derived phytochemicals reduce oxidative stress by activating Nrf2 by a ROS-independent mechanism and scavenging free radicals. Some examples are the organosulfur compound sulforaphane, found in cruciferous vegetables; kavalactones, found in kava shrubs; and puerarin, a major flavonoid from the root of *Pueraria lobata*. (Bergstrom et al. 2011) (Wruck et al. 2008; Zou et al. 2013). Also included are genistein and vitamin E (Xi et al. 2012), coenzyme Q10 (Choi et al. 2009), alpha-lipoic

acid (Suh et al. 2004), curcumin (Trujillo et al. 2013), resveratrol (Steele et al. 2013) (Kode et al. 2008), omega-3 fatty acids (Gao et al. 2007; Saw et al. 2013), and NAC (Ji et al. 2010).

3. Antioxidant chemical that can reduce oxidative stress by activating Nrf2 by a ROS-dependent mechanism. An example is L-carnitine (Zambrano et al. 2013).

A combination of selected agents from the above groups may optimally reduce oxidative stress, and thereby may reduce the risk of developing neurodegenerative disorders, and in combination with standard therapy, may improve the management of these conditions.

How to Reduce Chronic Inflammation and Glutamate Release

Some individual antioxidants from the groups above have been shown to reduce chronic inflammation (Abate et al. 2000; Devaraj et al. 2007; Fu et al. 2008; Lee et al. 2007; Peairs and Rankin 2008; Rahman et al. 2008; Suzuki, Aggarwal, and Packer 1992; Zhu et al. 2008). They have also been shown to prevent the release (Barger et al. 2007) and toxicity of glutamate (Schubert, Kimura, and Maher 1992; Sandhu et al. 2003). A combination of selected agents from the groups above may also optimally reduce chronic inflammation and the release of glutamate and its toxicity. In so doing, it may thereby reduce the risk of developing neurodegenerative diseases, and in combination with standard therapy, may improve the management of them.

PROBLEMS OF USING A SINGLE NUTRIENT IN CONCUSSIVE INJURY, PENETRATING TBI, AND PTSD

A few studies with individual polyphenolic compounds and one study with a preparation of micronutrients containing multiple dietary and endogenous antioxidants showed beneficial effects in animal models of TBI and troops exposed to concussive injury and war-related stressors. The fact that the patients with neurological injuries (concussion, penetrating TBI, and PTSD) have a high internal oxidative environment suggests that the administration of a single antioxidant would result in oxidation of administered antioxidant. It is well-known that an oxidized antioxidant acts as a pro-oxidant (like a free radical) that may not produce beneficial clinical outcomes. On the contrary, oxidized antioxidants are likely to continue to compound the effects of neurological damage after long-term consumption.

Previous studies in other chronic diseases, such as beta-carotene in male heavy smokers for reducing the risk of lung cancer, vitamin E in Alzheimer's disease (AD) for improving cognitive function and vitamin E in Parkinson's disease (PD) for improving the symptoms and as expected, produced inconsistent results varying from no effect as in PD (Shoulson 1998), to modest beneficial (Sano et al. 1997) or no effect as in AD (Farina et al. 2012), to harmful effects as in heavy male smokers (Albanes et al. 1995).

It is not possible to optimally reduce oxidative stress and chronic inflammation by the use of one or two antioxidants for improved management of concussive injury, penetrating TBI, and PTSD, because they may not increase the levels of all antioxidant enzymes as well as all dietary and endogenous antioxidants in the body at the same time. I therefore recommend, in combination with standard therapy, a preparation of micronutrients containing multiple dietary and endogenous antioxidants, vitamin D, B vitamins, certain minerals, and polyphenolic compounds (resveratrol, curcumin) and omega-3 fatty acids for the improved the management of concussive injury, penetrating TBI, and PTSD.

RATIONALE FOR USING MULTIPLE ANTIOXIDANTS IN CONCUSSIVE INJURY, PENETRATING TBI, AND PTSD*

The mechanisms of action of antioxidants in the proposed formulation are in part different from each other. Their distribution in various organs and cells, their affinity to various types of free radicals, and their biological half-lives are different. For example, beta-carotene (BC) is more effective in scavenging oxygen radicals than most other antioxidants. BC can perform certain biological functions that cannot be produced by vitamin A, and vitamin A can perform certain biological functions that cannot be performed by beta-carotene. It has been reported that BC treatment enhances the expression of the connexin gene that codes for a gap junction protein in mammalian fibroblasts in culture, whereas vitamin A treatment does not produce such an effect. Vitamin A can induce differentiation in certain normal and cancer cells, whereas BC and other carotenoids do not. Thus, BC and vitamin A have, in part, different functions in the body.

The gradient of oxygen pressure varies within the cells. Some antioxidants, such as vitamin E, are more effective as scavenger of free radicals in reduced oxygen pressure, whereas BC and vitamin A are more effective in higher atmospheric pressures.

Cells contain mostly water and some fat. Cellular components are distributed in the water and fat of the cells. Vitamin C is necessary to protect cellular components in the water portion of the cells, whereas carotenoids, vitamins A and vitamin E protect cellular components in the fat portion of the cells. Vitamin C also plays an important role in maintaining cellular levels of vitamin E by recycling oxidized form of vitamin E (acts as a pro-oxidant) to reduced form of vitamin E (acts as an antioxidant).

---

*The references for this section are described in a review (Prasad, Cole, and Prasad 2002).

The form of vitamin E used is also important for a micronutrient preparation. It has been established that d-alpha-tocopheryl succinate (vitamin E succinate) is the most effective form of vitamin E both *in vitro* and *in vivo*. This form of vitamin E is more soluble than alpha-tocopherol and enters cells more readily, therefore it's expected to cross the blood-brain barrier in greater amounts than alpha-tocopherol. We have reported that an oral ingestion of alpha-tocopheryl succinate (800 IU/day) in humans increased the plasma levels of not only alpha-tocopherol, but also of vitamin E succinate, suggesting that a portion of vitamin E succinate can be absorbed from the intestinal tract before conversion to alpha-tocopherol. This observation is important because the conventional assumption based on the studies in rodents has been that esterified forms of vitamin E, such as alpha-tocopheryl succinate, alpha-tocopheryl nicotinate, and alpha-tocopheryl acetate, can be absorbed from the intestinal tract only after they are converted to alpha-tocopherol form. Our preliminary data showed that this assumption may not be true for the absorption of vitamin E succinate in humans, provided the pool of alpha-tocopherol in the blood is saturated.

An endogenous (made in the body) antioxidant, glutathione, is effective in destroying H_2O_2 and superoxide anion (a form of free radical). However, oral supplementation with glutathione failed to significantly increase the plasma levels of glutathione in humans, suggesting that glutathione is completely destroyed in the intestine. Therefore, I propose to utilize n-acetylcysteine (NAC) and alpha-lipoic acid, which increase the cellular levels of glutathione by different mechanisms in a micronutrient preparation.

Other endogenous antioxidants and coenzyme Q10 may have some potential value in prevention and improved treatment of concussive injury, severe TBI, and PTSD. Coenzyme Q10 administration has been shown to improve clinical symptoms in other diseases such as in patients with mitochondrial encephalomyopathies (Chen, et al. 1997).

Since mitochondrial dysfunction is associated with most neurodegenerative diseases and since coenzyme Q10 is needed for the generation of ATP by mitochondria, it is essential to add this antioxidant to a micronutrient preparation. A study has shown that coenzyme Q10 scavenges peroxy radicals faster than alpha-tocopherol, and like vitamin C, can convert oxidized vitamin E to the reduced form of vitamin E, which acts as an antioxidant.

Excessive amounts of glutamate release may cause degeneration of the nerve cells in patients with concussive injury, severe TBI, and PTSD. Antioxidants reduced the release and toxicity of glutamate. Nicotinamide (vitamin B_3) attenuated glutamate-induced toxicity in nerve cells.

Although memory loss has been observed in patients who suffered the above-referenced neurological conditions, no study has been performed to improve cognitive function in these patients. However, in other neurodegenerative diseases, nicotinamide (vitamin B_3), which is also an inhibitor of histone deacetylase activity, can restore memory deficits in transgenic mice exhibiting the signs of Alzheimer's disease. Selenium is a co-factor of glutathione peroxidase, and Se-glutathione peroxidase acts as an antioxidant by increasing the intracellular level of glutathione.

In addition to dietary and endogenous antioxidants, B vitamins are also essential for normal brain function. Omega-3 fatty acids and curcumin were also added because clinical studies show some benefits in patients with penetrating TBI. Resveratrol was added because it has produced some beneficial effects in other neurodegenerative diseases.

Increased pro-inflammatory stimuli and oxidative stress cause microglia to release excessive amounts of glutamate, which not only maintain anxiety disorders through the NMDA receptor, but also contribute to neurodegeneration (Barger et al. 2007).

Release of glutamate was blocked by vitamin E (Barger et al. 2007). This could help in improving anxiety disorders. Indeed, an inhibitor of the NMDA receptor reduces anxiety (Davis et al. 2006), but is toxic.

Both vitamin E (Schubert, Kimura, and Maher 1992) and coenzyme Q10 (Sandhu et al. 2003) also protect against glutamate-induced neurotoxicity in cell-culture models.

Two recent clinical studies showed that supplementation with multivitamin preparations reduced cancer incidence by 10 percent in men (Gaziano et al. 2012) and improved clinical outcomes in patients with HIV/AIDS who were not taking medication (Baum et al. 2013).

CONCLUDING REMARKS

In this chapter we have discussed the properties and functions of antioxidants and polyphenolic compounds. As we have learned, certain antioxidants are consumed through the diet and others are made in the body. We have also determined that dietary and endogenous antioxidant chemicals and polyphenolic compounds reduce oxidative stress by directly scavenging free radicals. Other agents reduce oxidative stress by elevating antioxidant enzymes through the Nrf2/ARE pathway.

Several of these agents have a dual function because they can activate the ROS-independent Nrf2/ARE pathway for increasing antioxidant enzymes and elevate the levels of antioxidant chemicals. Thus it appears that selected agents from these groups of antioxidants at appropriate doses may be necessary for the prevention of neurodegenerative diseases. Unfortunately, as we know, clinical studies with antioxidants in a population at high risk of developing chronic disease have utilized a single antioxidant, or only a few. The results of these studies have been inconsistent.

A separate preparation of micronutrients, including dietary and endogenous antioxidants and certain polyphenolic compounds (curcumin and resveratrol) and omega-3 fatty acids, employed to reduce the risk of some chronic diseases, will be proposed in subsequent chapters. These agents are capable of reducing oxidative stress, chronic inflammation, and the release and toxicity of glutamate by increasing antioxidant enzyme levels through the Nrf2/ARE pathway as well as by scavenging free radicals directly.

Next we will turn our attention to the neurological problems that are the subject of this book: concussive injury, penetrating traumatic brain injury, and post-traumatic stress disorder, so that we may ascertain how to best treat these seemingly intractable conditions.

5 Concussive Injury

Causes, Symptoms, Incidence, and Costs

Concussive brain injury is also called mild traumatic brain injury (mild TBI); it can express in a mild, moderate, or severe form. A concussion typically occurs when there is a blow to the head or neck that causes the brain to move back and forth in an impactful way against the skull. There is no fracture of the skull in this form of brain injury. The word "concussion" derives from the Latin *concutere*, meaning "to shake violently."

Made of soft tissue and housed in spinal fluid that generally protects it, the brain undergoing a concussive injury is vulnerable, for a concussion is capable of doing serious damage to the brain, including damaging its blood vessels. A concussive injury may also effect immediate and transient changes in brain function, which may include temporary loss of memory, confusion, poor balance and reflexes, and hearing loss.

This chapter briefly describes the causes, symptoms, incidence, and costs of concussive injury. In addition, this chapter also describes studies done on the role of increased oxidative stress, chronic inflammation, and glutamate release as they pertain to concussive injury.

CAUSES OF CONCUSSIVE INJURY

Concussive injury occurs when the brain is rocked violently back and forth within the skull following a blow to the head or neck such as that observed in contact sports like football and soccer. Concussive injury also occurs in troops who are exposed to a blast pressure wave, such as following detonation of an explosive device. Among civilians, falls and crashes involving automobiles, motorcycles, and bicycles can cause concussive injury.

SYMPTOMS OF CONCUSSIVE INJURY

The major acute physical symptoms of a concussive injury include transient confusion, disorientation and loss of consciousness, headache, dizziness, nausea, blurred vision, uneven gait, insomnia, and fatigue. The cognitive dysfunctions such as memory loss, attention deficit, and lack of concentration and behavioral abnormalities appear as late effects of concussion. Behavioral changes include irritability, depression, fear and anxiety, loss of emotional control, and problems with relationships.

INCIDENCE OF CONCUSSIVE INJURY

The Center for Disease Control and Prevention (CDC, 2012) estimates that 1.7 million people in the United States sustain a traumatic brain injury (TBI) annually from all causes. Of these injuries, approximately 75 percent of them are concussive injuries. Let's look at some of these populations—athletes, soldiers, and civilians—among which concussive injuries occur, beginning with professional athletes, specifically, members of the National Football League.

National Football League (NFL) Players
Between 2002 and 2007, 152 players in the NFL suffered from repeat concussions (Casson et al. 2011). The positions that have the highest

incidence of repeat concussion include the defensive secondary, kick unit, running back, and linebacker. About 7.6 percent of all repeat concussions occurred within 2 weeks of the prior concussion. More than half of the players with repeat concussion were removed from play.

High School and College Athletes

Among young people ages 15–24 years, sports are second to motor vehicle crashes as the leading cause of TBI. Football accounted for more than half of all concussions in the boys. Of the sports that the girls played, soccer was accorded the highest proportion of concussive injury. The incidence of concussive injury increased 4-fold between the years 1998–2008.

Another study has estimated that about 300,000 sports-related concussive injuries occur among high school and college athletes per year in various high schools and colleges. Concussive injury represented 8.9 percent of all high school athletic injuries and 5.8 percent of all college athletic injuries (Gessel et al. 2007). The rates of concussions were highest among athletes playing football and soccer. The rate of concussive injury was higher in girls than in boys.

The number of U.S. students participating in high school and college sports is increasing. In 2004–2005 more than 385,000 college students participated in sports and in 2005–2006 more than seven million high school students were likewise engaged. According to the National Federation of State High School Associations, in 2008–2009 about 7.5 million high school students participated in sports. In addition, the trend of participating in competitive sports at a younger age is increasing. Thus, the number of individuals with concussive injury is expected to increase in future.

Veterans of Foreign Wars

Among U.S. veterans returning from military conflicts in Iraq and Afghanistan, traumatic brain injury (TBI) represents one of the major injuries. The prevalence of TBI ranges from 15 to 20 percent of troops operating in the combat zone. It has been estimated that 85 percent of the TBIs are mild concussions (MacGregor et al. 2011). The majority of these concussions were due to exposure to blasts, with most of the troops experiencing exposure to multiple blasts. About 20 percent of the soldiers were exposed to a second blast within 2 weeks of the first, and 87 percent of them were exposed to a second blast within 3 months of the original explosion.

Civilians

In the civilian population, falls, motor vehicle accidents, the striking of stationary or moving objects, and assaults involving the head contribute to concussive injury, or mild to severe TBI (CDC, Traumatic Brain Injury and Causes, 2012). Table 5.1 details the incidence of concussive injury in civilians. Falls are the major causes of concussive injury among children up to the age of 14 and among adults age 65 or older.

TABLE 5.1. CONDITIONS CONTRIBUTING TO THE INCIDENCE OF CONCUSSIVE INJURY IN CIVILIANS

Conditions	Percent of Concussive Injury
Fall	35.2
Motor vehicle accident	17.3
Being struck by moving/ stationary objects	16.5
Assaults	10
Other unknown factors	21

COSTS OF CONCUSSIVE INJURY

The direct and indirect medical costs (loss of productivity) of mild TBI or concussive injury each year is estimated to be $17 billion (CDC, Traumatic Brain Injury and Causes, 2012). Given these enormous financial impacts on society, what is currently being done to mitigate the incidence of concussion? Numerous studies have been undertaken to determine more about this troubling injury, in the hopes that its occurrence may be reduced. Let's look at some of these very important studies next.

THE EFFECT OF CONCUSSIVE INJURY ON BRAIN FUNCTION: THE HUMAN STUDIES

Human studies on the effects of concussion on the brain have revealed that the precipitating injury may spawn a whole host of other problems. Some of these findings are included here.

Deformation of the brain structure may occur after the primary head acceleration (Viano et al. 2005).

Damage to the mid-brain correlated with memory and cognitive problems following concussion. The major changes after concussion included impairment of temporary loss of memory, confusion, poor balance and reflexes, hearing loss, cognitive dysfunction, and abnormal behavior (Rapoport et al. 2005; van Donkelaar et al. 2005; Halterman et al. 2006).

Among professional football players, an early onset of dementia may be initiated by repetitive concussions (Guskiewicz et al. 2005; Gottshall et al. 2003).

Balance problems are also considered one of the major health issues following mild TBI (Gottshall et al. 2003; Viano et al. 2006).

In a clinical study of 1,044 members of the National Football League Retired Players Association, the effect of one or more concussions on the incidence of depression 9 years after the incident was evaluated. This was done by utilizing the General Health Survey Questionnaire (Kerr et al. 2012). The results showed that 10.2 percent of participating players had depression, which increased with the number of concussions experienced, as compared with those retired players who reported no concussions. An increase in concussion-induced depression was independent of depression induced by other causes.

In another clinical study of 2,552 retired professional football players with an average age of 45.8, the effect of concussions on the risk of developing mild cognitive dysfunction and Alzheimer's disease was evaluated (Guskiewicz et al. 2005). The results showed that retired players with 3 or more concussions had a 5-fold prevalence of mild cognitive dysfunction and a 3-fold increase in significant memory loss compared to those retired players who did not suffer concussions. The onset of Alzheimer's disease among the retired players appeared earlier than among the general American population.

In a study of college football players, it was found that players with a history of previous concussion were more likely to have future concussions than those with no history of concussion. About 85.2 percent of retired players reported headache that lasted up to 82 hours. If one had suffered from a previous concussion, recovery time was slower (Guskiewicz et al. 2003).

Increased risk of chronic traumatic encephalopathy (CTE) remains one of the measurable health concerns of repeat concussion. In a study of high school football players, it was found that repetitive blows to the head are cumulative, and that repeated subconcussive blows can cause CTE and neurophysiological abnormalities (Breedlove et al. 2012).

Concussion can cause a decline in motor and cognitive function and an increased risk of Alzheimer's disease in young athletes. Animal models of TBI have shown that impaired learning ability was related to the suppression of synaptic activity. In humans, single or repeated concussion can cause lifelong or cumulative enhancement of gamma-aminobutyric acid (GABA)-mediated suppression of synapse function. It has been reported that repeated concussion induced persistent elevation of GABA-mediated inhibition of synaptic activity in the motor cortex (De Beaumont et al. 2012). These changes are considered important factors contributing to impaired brain functions.

In a clinical study of 79 concussed college athletes, a computerized neuropsychological test was given during the preseason and on the second and eighth day after a concussion had occurred. The results showed that concussed female athletes performed significantly worse than concussed male athletes on visual memory tasks (Covassin, Schatz, and Swanik 2007). Male athletes were more likely to report symptoms of vomiting and sadness than female athletes. The analysis of performance data further revealed that at 2 days after injury, 58 percent of concussed athletes exhibited a decline in performance and an increase in other symptoms whereas at 8 days after concussions, 30 percent continue to show one or more changes in neuropsychological tests.

In another study, an anonymous mental health survey was performed on 1,502 American Army soldiers 4 to 6 months after they had returned from deployment to Iraq or Afghanistan (Wilk et al. 2012). The results showed that 17 percent of soldiers reported a mild TBI during their previous deployment, and 59 percent of these soldiers suffered more than one mild TBI. After adjusting for post-traumatic stress disorder (PTSD), depression, and other factors, multiple mild TBI with loss of consciousness increased the risk of headache compared to those who had only one mild TBI.

Mild TBI is also associated with an increased incidence of PTSD. The similarity in some of the symptoms between mild TBI and PTSD makes it difficult to distinguish them when evaluating for the treatment of these brain dysfunctions. A review of 3 large studies on the frequency of mild TBI and PTSD in veterans of Iraq and Afghanistan showed that frequencies of mild TBI/PTSD were from 5–7 percent. Among those with mild TBI, frequencies of PTSD ranged from 33–39 percent (Carlson et al. 2011).

Studies of functional and metabolic imaging suggest that abnormalities in the electric responses, metabolic balance, and oxygen consumption in neurons exist several months after concussion (Ellemberg et al. 2009).

BIOCHEMICAL DEFECTS IN
CONCUSSIVE INJURY

Studies primarily on animal models of concussion suggest that increased oxidative stress, chronic inflammation, and glutamate release play a central role in the progression of concussive injury. These studies are described here.

Evidence of Increased Oxidative Stress in Mild TBI (Concussive Injury)

Evidence for increased oxidative stress is derived from the levels of markers of oxidative damage that are elevated after concussion, and from antioxidants that are reduced after concussion. It has been reported that elevated levels of oxidized proteins, reduced levels of superoxide dismutase (SOD), and silent information regulator-2 (Sir2) were observed after a mild TBI in the hippocampus of rats (Wu et al. 2010). In addition, poor performance by these animals was associated with reduced levels of brain-derived neurotrophic factor (BDNF). BDNF facilitates synaptic function and supports learning ability. A feeding diet supplemented with vitamin E for 4 weeks before a mild TBI prevented impairment in learning ability and the above-referenced biochemical defects in these rats. These results suggest that increased oxidative stress may impair the learning ability of animals with a mild TBI.

In a transgenic mouse model of Alzheimer's disease, repetitive concussive brain injury increased the levels of brain lipid peroxidation, accelerated beta-amyloid deposition, and caused learning deficits. A feeding diet supplemented with vitamin E for 4 weeks before the occurrence of mild TBI prevented lipid peroxidation, impairment in learning ability, and reduction in the levels of BDNF in these transgenic mice (Conte et al. 2004).

It has been reported that a high-fat diet decreased hippocampal plasticity and cognitive function by reducing BDNF in rats with mild TBI (Wu et al. 2003).

A feeding diet supplemented with curcumin, which exhibits antioxidant and anti-inflammatory activities, prevented oxidative stress, restored BDNF, and improved synaptic function and cognitive function in rats with mild TBI (Wu, Ying, and Gomez-Pinilla 2006).

Similar results were obtained by a feeding diet supplemented with the omega-3 fatty acids docosahexaenoic acid (DHA) prior to inducing a mild TBI in rats (Wu, Ying, and Gomez-Pinilla 2011).

Repetitive concussive injury increased the levels of markers of oxidative damage, such as malondialdehyde (MDA), nitrite, nitrate, and decreased ascorbic acid and glutathione levels in rats. These biochemical changes were observed in rats in which mild TBI was delivered 1, 2, or 3 days after the first one. However, if the time interval between the first one and second one was 5 days, biochemical markers of oxidative and nitrosylative stress were nearly control levels (Tavazzi et al. 2007). This suggests that the greater time interval between two concussions may allow recovery of some damage.

■ ■ ■

As regards human studies, none have been performed on changes in the markers of oxidative damage or the levels of antioxidants following concussive injury in active or retired football players. However, it should be pointed out that during a typical game, football players are exposed to excessive amounts of oxygen.

Normally, about 20 percent of respired oxygen is used by the brain. Mitochondria utilize oxygen to generate energy, and free radicals are produced during this process. About 2 percent of unused oxygen leaks out of mitochondria, which produces approximately 20 billion molecules of superoxide anions and hydrogen peroxide per cell per day. Thus, it's likely that during a game, when excessive amounts of oxygen are used, the brain may be exposed to higher levels of oxidative stress, which may overwhelm endogenous defense systems. This may enhance the damaging effects of concussion.

Evidence of Inflammation in Mild TBI (Concussive Injury)

In Animal Studies

Only one animal study has been performed to date to evaluate the role of inflammation in the development and progression of concussive injury. Acute and chronic inflammation occurs in response to damage caused by concussion. Rats exposed to repetitive concussions (1, 3, or 5 times) spaced 5 days apart displayed increased anxiety and depressionlike behaviors, short- and long-term cognitive dysfunction, chronic inflammation, and damage to the cortex (Shultz et al. 2012).

In Human Studies

Time-dependent changes in inflammatory cellular response in human cortical contusion were investigated during the first 30 weeks following a blunt head injury (Hausmann et al. 1999). The results showed that CD-15 (3-fucosyl-N-acertyl-lactosamine)-labeled granulocytes were detected as early as 10 minutes after brain injury. In addition, increased numbers of mononuclear leukocytes labeled with LCA (leukocyte common antigen), CD-3, and UCHL-1, a clone of CD45RO that is an isoform of LCA, were detected at 1.1 days, 2 days, and 3.7 days after cortical contusions.

In another study, time-dependent alterations in inflammatory responses of 12 consecutive patients undergoing surgery for brain contusions 3 hours to 5 days after the precipitating trauma were determined (Holmin et al. 1998). If the inflammatory responses were determined in less than 24 hours after the injury, they were limited to vascular margination of polymorphonuclear cells. In patients undergoing surgery 3–5 days after injury, an extensive inflammatory reaction consisting of monocyte/macrophages, reactive microglia, polymorphonuclear cells, and CD-4 and CD-8-labeled T lymphocytes was observed. The human lymphocyte antigen-DQ was expressed on reactive microglia and infiltrating leukocytes later on. These inflammatory cells that appear following contusions may produce several potentially harmful effects, including acute and long-term degeneration of nerve cells.

The expression of pro- and anti-inflammatory cytokines released by microglia cells was determined after surgery (Holmin and Hojeberg 2004). The results showed that in patients undergoing surgery less than 24 hours after injury, an elevated expression of the pro-inflammatory cytokines interleukin-1 beta (IL-1 beta), IL-6, interferon-gamma (INF-gamma), and the anti-inflammatory cytokine IL-4 was present. In patients undergoing surgery 3–5 days after injury, the expression of IL-4 was lower compared to those who had been operated on earlier. However, the expression of IL-1beta and IFN-gamma remained high compared to IL-6. The persistence of pro-inflammatory cytokines could cause degeneration of nerve cells after concussive injury.

Autopsied Samples of the Brain in Concussive Injury in Human Studies

In studies on autopsied brain samples from 24 patients who had TBI and 5 healthy individuals brains, changes in CD-14, a pattern-recognition receptor of the immune system, were investigated (Beschorner et al. 2002). In healthy brains, CD-14 expressed constitutively in perivascular cells, but not in parenchymal cells. However, after TBI, expression of CD-14 in perivascular cells and parenchymal cells reached maximal levels within 4–8 days and remained elevated until weeks after injury. These results suggest that increased expression of CD-14 is one of the major responses of acute inflammatory reaction in the brain following TBI.

Evidence of Increased Glutamate Release in Concussive Injury in Animal Studies

Glutamate is highly toxic to nerve cells in the brain. Mild traumatic injury (concussive brain injury) can cause cognitive and emotional dysfunction and increase the risk for the development of anxiety disorders, including post-traumatic stress disorder (PTSD), which is commonly observed among veterans of foreign wars.

Glutamate receptor N-methy-D-aspartate (NMDA) in the amygdala appears to regulate fear and anxiety. In a rat model of mild TBI, the levels of NMDA receptors in the amygdala increased. In addition, gamma-aminobutyric acid (GABA)-related inhibition decreased in the amygdala and the hippocampus (Reger et al. 2012). These results suggest excitatory conditions (presence of increased levels of glutamate) created by an elevation of NMDA receptor levels and a decrease in GABA activity, which may increase the risk of developing fear and anxiety. It appears that following concussive brain injury, excessive amounts of glutamate are released that can cause a massive efflux of K+ ions and an increased accumulation of lactate. This was confirmed by the fact that administration of ouabain, an inhibitor of Na+/K+-ATPase, before injury reduced lactate accumulation. Thus, increased levels of glutamate may be present after concussion.

Evidence of Molecular Changes in the Brain in Concussive Injury in Animal Studies

The expression of oncogenes c-myc and c-fos was elevated in rat brains after concussion (Fang, Wang, and Wang 2006; Wang, Li, and Hu 2003).

In addition, expression of nuclear factor kappaB (NF-kappaB) was elevated in the cortex of a human contused brain (Hang et al. 2006).

The fact that antioxidants reduced expression of c-myc oncogene (Prasad, Cohrs, and Sharma 1990) and activation of NF-KappaB (Shen, Zhang, and Zhang 2003) further suggests that supplementation with antioxidants may reduce acute and long-term term adverse effects of concussive injury on brain functions. The levels of inducible nitric oxide synthase (iNOS) in human neurons, macrophages, neutrophils, astrocytes, and oligodendrocytes increased within 6 hours after brain trauma, and peaked at about 8–23 hours (Gahm, Holmin, and Mathiesen 2002). Increased levels of iNOS can generate excessive amounts of NO, which can form peroxynitrite that is very toxic to the nerve cells in the brain.

CONCLUDING REMARKS

Brain injuries are as old as humanity, for mankind has always engaged in warfare, whether by using stones, spears, bow and arrows, or bombs, missiles, and IEDs. Only recently, however, has this form of injury drawn significant attention from doctors, scientists, and the public. This is due to the fact that current medical interventions soon after injury have produced increased numbers of survivors, and also because serious neurological problems such as cognitive dysfunction and other forms of neurological disorders are observed as late effects of concussions.

Current strategies for reducing the adverse impacts of concussion on brain function have focused on the development of physical protection in order to protect the skull from the impacts of concussion. In the case of football players, the introduction of newer football helmets appears to have lowered the risk of concussion by about 10–20 percent (Viano et al. 2006), which appears very low.

Most human studies of concussions have focused on incidence, cost, and the mental disorders that are associated with concussion, which includes cognitive dysfunction and changes in behavior. A few studies have investigated changes in the brain structure and in markers of oxidative damage and chronic inflammation and glutamate release following concussive injury—primarily in animal models. From these studies, it appears that an increase in oxidative stress, chronic inflammation, and glutamate release may contribute to the development and progression of mental disorders following concussive injury.

Currently, treatments involving medications and other complementary therapeutic approaches are not satisfactory. Thus concussive brain injury remains a major health risk for professional football players (Guskiewicz et al. 2000; Levy et al. 2004) and for U.S. soldiers, veterans, and others who continue to suffer from the consequences of concussion on brain function.

6

Treating and Managing Concussive Injury with Vitamins and Antioxidants

As described in the previous chapter, increased oxidative stress, chronic inflammation, and glutamate release are major biochemical defects that initiate damage in the brain following concussion. Therefore, reducing these biochemical defects would protect the brain from further damage following concussive injury, and would complement protection provided by physical devices.

In order to optimally reduce oxidative stress, chronic inflammation, and glutamate release and its toxicity, it's essential to increase levels of dietary and endogenous antioxidant chemicals as well as antioxidant enzymes by the activation of the Nrf2/ARE pathway at the same time. This goal can't be achieved by the use of a single antioxidant. Therefore, I have proposed a preparation of micronutrients containing multiple dietary and endogenous antioxidants and certain polyphenolic compounds (curcumin and resveratrol), and omega-3 fatty acids that would activate a nuclear transcriptional factor-2 (Nrf2)/ ARE (antioxidant response element) pathway and increase the levels of antioxidant enzymes and antioxidant chemicals in the body at the same time. Unfortunately, only a few animal studies on the role of individual antioxidants in reducing the impact of concussion on brain functions are currently available (chapter 5).

This chapter proposes a novel concept of PAMARA (protection as much as reasonably achievable), which includes protection of the skull by physical devices and protection of the brain tissue by a preparation of micronutrients. This chapter also provides scientific rationale for using a preparation of micronutrients for reducing the acute and long-term adverse effects of concussive injury in a most effective manner.

THE CONCEPT OF PAMARA

The concept of PAMARA (protection as much as reasonably achievable), involves protecting the skull by physical devices and protecting brain tissue by reducing oxidative stress and chronic inflammation by supplementation with a preparation of micronutrients that contain multiple dietary and endogenous antioxidants and omega-3 fatty acids. However, the concept of PAMARA has not been tested in concussive injury. Although some studies have investigated the efficacy of physical devices in reducing the risk of concussion, the efficacy of proposed micronutrient formulations for mitigation of brain concussive injury has not been tested on high school or college athletes. Nor has it been tested on professional athletes.

Be that as it may, the proposed micronutrient recommendations can be adopted by those individuals who are exposed to or who have already been exposed to concussive injury. This should be done in consultation with one's physician or health care professional. It's expected that the proposed recommendations, when used before sporting events, may complement physical protection devices to reduce damage to the brain following concussion. When used *after* concussive injury in combination with standard care, it may reduce the risk of developing abnormal brain function, including cognitive dysfunction and aberrant behavior.

THE EFFECT OF A SINGLE ANTIOXIDANT IN STUDIES OF CONCUSSIVE INJURY IN ANIMAL STUDIES

Vitamin E

A feeding diet supplemented with vitamin E for 4 weeks before a mild TBI prevented impairment in learning ability and biochemical defects such as increased levels of oxidized proteins, and reduced levels of superoxide dismutase (SOD) and BDNF (brain-derived neurotrophic factor) in the hippocampus of rats (Wu et al. 2010).

A feeding diet supplemented with vitamin E for 4 weeks prior to mild repetitive TBI prevented lipid peroxidation, impairment in learning ability, accelerated beta-amyloid deposition, and reduction in the levels of BDNF in a transgenic mouse model of Alzheimer's disease (Conte et al. 2004).

Curcumin and Omega-3 Fatty Acids

As we articulated in the last chapter, a diet that included curcumin prevented oxidative stress, restored BDNF, and improved synaptic function and cognitive function in rats with mild TBI (Wu, Ying, and Gomez-Pinilla 2006). This is because curcumin exhibits antioxidant and anti-inflammatory activities and activates Nrf2.

Also as articulated in the last chapter but which bears repeating here, supplementing the diet with the omega-3 fatty acid, docosahexaenoic acid (DHA) prior to inducing a mild TBI in rats produced comparable outcomes (Wu, Ying, and Gomez-Pinilla 2011).

THE EFFECT OF MULTIPLE ANTIOXIDANTS IN TROOPS EXPOSED TO CONCUSSIVE INJURY

A commercial formulation of multiple micronutrients was tested in a clinical study in troops returning from Iraq with mild to moderate

TBI. These patients had not developed symptoms of PTSD, because they were recruited for the study after a few weeks of exposure to blasts and other traumatic events. Thirty-four patients with post-traumatic dizziness were admitted to the Naval Medical Center San Diego Clinic over a 2-month period of time and agreed to participate in the study under the supervision of Dr. Michael Hoffer and his colleagues (Gottshall 2006).

All patients had received their injury 3 to 20 weeks prior to admission, and they received identical treatment consisting of medical therapy (for any migraines), supportive care, steroids, and vestibular rehabilitation therapy. Fifteen of the 34 patients also received a dose of an antioxidant and micronutrient formula (2 capsules by mouth twice a day). At the onset of therapy all patients were evaluated by outcome measures that included the Sensory Organization Test (SOT) by Computerized Dynamic Posturography (CDP), the Dynamic Gait Index (DGI), the Activities Balance Confidence (ABC) scale, the Dizziness Handicap Index (DHI), the Vestibular Disorders Activities of Daily Living (VADL) score, and the Balance Scoring System (BESS) test. The study was carried out for 12 weeks. The therapist who graded these outcomes and performed the testing was blinded as to whether the patient was receiving antioxidant therapy or not. The pretrial test scores did not differ significantly between the 2 groups on any of the tests.

Both groups of patients showed trends toward significant improvement on all tests after the 12 weeks of therapy, but the combination treatment trend was stronger than that of the standard therapy alone group. After only 4 weeks, the SOT score by CDP was 78 for the antioxidant group as compared to 63 for the non-antioxidant group. This difference was statistically significant at the $P < 0.05$ level. The improvement noted by the antioxidant group on the other tests was also greater than the non-antioxidant group, although these differences did not reach statistical significance because of the short trial period and small sample size.

This study should be expanded using a randomized, double-blind and placebo-control clinical study design in which the efficacy of the proposed multiple micronutrients preparation would be tested in soldiers returning from combat theaters exhibiting mild to moderate traumatic brain injury or any sign of mental disorders such as anxiety, fear, and depression.

PROPOSED PREVENTION STRATEGIES IN CONCUSSIVE INJURY

Primary Prevention of Concussive Injury

The purpose of primary prevention is to protect athletes from developing concussion-related brain damage. The active players of sports, such as football players, constitute an excellent population in which to study primary prevention. Since excessive amounts of free radicals and chronic inflammation are generated during a sporting event, and more so following a concussive injury, reducing these biochemical defects appears to be a logical choice for the primary prevention of concussive injury.

Recommendations for Primary Prevention of Concussive Injury, Penetrating TBI, and PTSD

In providing an overview of guidelines regarding recommendations for the primary prevention of concussive injury, we will extend our remarks to include penetrating TBI and PTSD as well, given that the general guidelines as regards ingredients, dose-schedule, and toxicity are the same for all three groups.

Additionally, it should be noted that the effectiveness of *all* of the proposed micronutrient formulations contained in this book and recommended by its author, for both primary prevention and secondary prevention of concussive injury, penetrating TBI, and PTSD, should be tested by well-designed clinical studies. In the meantime, the specific protocols may be adopted by the respective parties at risk or those who suffer from any of the debilitating effects of concussive injury, penetrating TBI, or PTSD, in consultation with their health care providers.

Ingredients: The selected combination of nontoxic agents include vitamin A (retinyl palmitate), vitamin E (both d-alpha-tocopherol and d-alpha-tocopheryl succinate), natural mixed carotenoids, vitamin C (calcium ascorbate), vitamin D, B vitamins, selenium, coenzyme Q10, alpha-lipoic acid, n-acetylcysteine (NAC), L-carnitine, omega-3 fatty acids, resveratrol, and curcumin. This combination of agents was selected because they function to optimally reduce oxidative stress and chronic inflammation by activating the Nrf2/ARE pathway without ROS stimulation, and by directly scavenging free radicals.

Dose-schedule: Most clinical studies with antioxidants in chronic diseases have utilized a once-a-day dose-schedule. Taking vitamins and antioxidants once a day can create large fluctuations of their levels in the body. This is due to the fact that the biological half-lives of vitamins and antioxidants markedly vary, depending upon their lipid or water solubility. A 2-fold difference in the levels of vitamin E succinate can produce marked alterations in the expression profiles of several genes in nerve cells in culture. Therefore, taking a multivitamin preparation once a day may produce a large fluctuation in the levels of micronutrients in the body, which could potentially cause genetic stress in the cells that may compromise the effectiveness of the vitamin supplementation after long-term consumption.

Therefore, I recommend taking the proposed preparation of micronutrients twice a day in order to reduce fluctuations in the levels of gene expressions in the body. Such a dose-schedule may improve the effectiveness of the proposed micronutrient preparation in reducing the development of concussive injury, severe TBI, and PTSD. The daily doses can be divided in two, with half taken in the morning and half in the evening, preferably with a meal.

Toxicity Concerns: The proposed formulation of micronutrients has no iron, copper, manganese, or heavy metals (vanadium, zirconium, or molybdenum). Iron and copper are not added because they are known to interact with vitamin C to generate excessive amounts of free radicals. In addition, iron and copper are absorbed more readily in the presence of antioxidants than in the absence of antioxidants. Therefore, it is possible that prolonged consumption of these trace minerals in the presence of antioxidants may increase the levels of free iron or copper stores in the body, because there are no significant mechanisms of excretion of iron among men of all ages and women after menopause. Increased stores of free iron or copper may increase the risk of some human chronic diseases.

Heavy metals are not added because prolonged consumption of these metals may increase their levels in the body, because there is no significant mechanism for excretion of these metals from the body. High levels of these metals are considered neurotoxic. Antioxidants, B vitamins, and certain polyphenolic compounds (curcumin and resveratrol) used in the proposed micronutrient preparation are considered safe. Antioxidants at doses higher than those that are recommended for the proposed micronutrient preparation have been consumed by the U.S. population for decades without significant toxicity. (All ingredients present in the proposed micronutrient come under category of "Food Supplement," and therefore, do not require FDA approval for their use.)

Secondary Prevention of Concussive Injury
The purpose of secondary prevention is to stop or slow the progression of concussive injury in those individuals who are exposed

to repeated concussions but have not developed any clinical signs of neurological disorders. As we have learned, following a concussion, the levels of free radicals, chronic inflammation, and glutamate release—which play an important role in the progression of concussive injury—are increased. Therefore, reducing these biochemical defects may be a very viable strategy to employ to retard the progression of concussive injury.

Recommended Micronutrients in Secondary Prevention of Concussive Injury

The doses of all ingredients recommended for high school and college athletes and professional football players are listed in tables 6.1 and 6.2, respectively, on the next pages.

The recommended micronutrient preparation for reducing the effects of concussion on brain function among professional/college athletes are similar to those of high school athletes (table 6.2) except for higher doses of certain ingredients.

Diet and Lifestyle Recommendations for Concussive Injury

I recommend following the guidelines of the coaching staff's nutritional expert before and during the game. Retired players who have suffered concussions during the game, civilians who have had accidents or veterans of foreign wars should follow a balanced diet low in fat and high in fiber (from fruits and vegetables). Lifestyle recommendations include stopping tobacco smoking as well as use of tobacco products; reducing physical and mental stress by taking vacations, performing meditation or yoga; and consistently getting three to five days of moderate exercise per week.

TABLE 6.1. MICRONUTRIENT FORMULATION FOR HIGH SCHOOL ATHLETES (DAILY DOSES)*

Vitamin A (retinyl palmitate)	3,000 IU
Natural vitamin E	200 IU (d-alpha-tocopheryl succinate 100 IU) (d-alpha-tocopheryl acetate 100 IU)
Vitamin C (calcium ascorbate)	500 mg
Vitamin D_3 (cholecalciferol)	500 IU
Vitamin B_1 (thiamine mononitrate)	4 mg
Vitamin B_2 (riboflavin)	5 mg
Vitamin B_3 (nicotinamide)	50 mg
Vitamin B_6 (pyridoxine hydrochloride)	2 mg
Folic acid (as folate)	400 mcg
Vitamin B_{12} (methylcobalamln)	20 mcg
Biotin	200 mcg
Pantothenic acid (calcium pantothenate)	5 mg
Zinc glycinate	15 mg
Selenium (seleno-L-methionine)	100 mcg
N-acetylcysteine (NAC)	proprietary amount[†]
Coenzyme Q10	proprietary amount
Alpha-lipoic acid	proprietary amount
L-carnitine	proprietary amount
Natural carotenoids	proprietary amount
Resveratrol	proprietary amount
Curcumin	proprietary amount
Omega-3 fatty acids	proprietary amount

*Total capsules per day can be taken orally, half in the morning and half in the evening with a meal.
†Total amounts of antioxidants and herbal products come to 520 mg

TABLE 6.2. MICRONUTRIENT FORMULATION FOR COLLEGE/ PROFESSIONAL ATHLETES (DAILY DOSES)*

Vitamin A (retinyl palmitate)	3,000 IU
Natural vitamin E	400 IU (d-alpha-tocopheryl succinate 250 IU) (d-alpha-tocopheryl acetate 150 IU)
Vitamin C (calcium ascorbate)	1,000 mg
Vitamin D$_3$ (cholecalciferol)	1,000 IU
Vitamin B$_1$ (thiamine mononitrate)	10 mg
Vitamin B$_2$ (riboflavin)	4 mg
Vitamin B$_3$ (nicotinamide)	100 mg
Vitamin B$_6$ (pyridoxine hydrochloride)	4 mg
Folic acid (as folate)	400 mcg
Vitamin B$_{12}$ (methyl-cobalamln)	100 mcg
Biotin	200 mcg
Pantothenic acid (calcium pantothenate)	15 mg
Zinc glycinate	5 mg
Selenium (seleno-L-methionine)	100 mcg
N-acetylcysteine (NAC)	proprietary amount[†]
Coenzyme Q10	proprietary amount
Alpha-lipoic acid	proprietary amount
L-carnitine	proprietary amount
Natural carotenoids	proprietary amount
Resveratrol	proprietary amount
Curcumin	proprietary amount
Omega-3 fatty acids	proprietary amount

*Total capsules per day can be taken orally, half in the morning and half in the evening with a meal
†Total amounts of antioxidants and herbal products come to 1,585 mg

CONCLUDING REMARKS

Concussive injury is a serious condition that affects increasing numbers of individuals each and every year. Its long-term health risks include serious mental disorders such as cognitive dysfunction and abnormal behavior (fear, anxiety, anger, and suicidal tendencies), all of which are being observed at elevated rates among retired professional football players and veterans of foreign wars.

For professional athletes and soldiers, concussive injury remains a major health risk. It also remains a major health risk for the civilian population who may undergo a concussive injury as a result of a fall, or an automobile accident or other damaging event. This reality, coupled with the fact that current standards of care for concussion are unsatisfactory, presents a rather grim outlook for its prognosis.

Physical protection devices continue to be utilized in its prevention and in my view, this is a sound approach, but one that should be combined with therapeutic supplementation with micronutrients to further protect the at-risk individual.

The standard therapy for the management of late adverse effects of concussion on brain function remains unsatisfactory. This is due to the fact that standard therapy does not affect the levels of oxidative stress, chronic inflammation, or glutamate release and its toxicity that contribute to the progression of concussive injury. Reducing these biochemical defects simultaneously in combination with standard therapy, and the wearing of protective headgear, would reduce the progression of concussive injury, and would also improve the management of it.

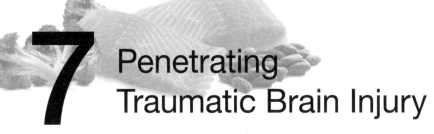

7 Penetrating Traumatic Brain Injury

Symptoms and Long-Term Effects, Incidence, and Costs

Penetrating traumatic brain injury (TBI) occurs when an object penetrates through the skull and damages the brain. This can be caused by vehicle crashes, gunshot wounds to the head, or exposure to explosions and combat-related injuries. Progression of damage in penetrating TBI occurs in three phases. The first phase involves injury to the brain tissue that cannot be reversed, because the damaged tissue is irreversibly lost.

The second phase of injury continues for days to weeks after the initial event and eventually leads to mental disorders and death of nerve cells. During this period, administration of appropriate agents may slow down the progression of the damage.

The third phase of penetrating TBI appears as delayed behavioral abnormalities, which depend upon the intial areas of the brain damaged. These may include memory loss, PTSD, and other behavioral defects.

There are two categories of penetrating traumatic brain injury: mild and severe. If the injury results in a loss of consciousness and/or confusion that lasts for less than thirty minutes, the injury is deemed to be mild. A loss of consciousness lasting over half an hour and/or memory loss lasting more than twenty-four hours are hallmarks of severe penetrating TBI. Advanced medical technologies have increased the survival rates of individuals with penetrating TBI, placing more individuals in long-term rehabilitative care.

This chapter briefly describes the causes, symptoms, incidence, costs, and major biochemical defects that contribute to the progression of penetrating TBI. It presents extensive data to show that increased oxidative stress, acute and chronic inflammation, and excessive release of glutamate into the extracellular fluid of the brain play an important role in the progression of acute and late phases of penetrating TBI.

Concussive injury in the brain occurs without injury to the skull. It is also called mild TBI. In contrast to concussive injury, penetrating TBI occurs with injury to the skull. Both forms of TBI can occur as mild or severe.

CAUSES OF PENETRATING TBI

Penetrating TBI occurs when an object penetrates the skull and damages the brain; this damage may be confined to a small area of the brain or be much more extensive. Among U.S. soldiers deployed to war, blasts, IEDs, vehicular crashes, and other combat-related injuries are the main causes of the increased incidence of penetrating TBI. Among civilians, transportation accidents involving automobiles, motorcycles, bicycles, and pedestrians, as well as gunshot wounds to the head are major causes of penetrating TBI. A penetrating TBI is a serious and life-threatening injury that requires emergency medical attention and care.

IMMEDIATE SYMPTOMS OF SEVERE TBI

The acute symptoms of severe TBI, which appear soon after injury, may include the following:

1. heavy bleeding from the head
2. bleeding from the ears
3. difficulty breathing
4. seizure
5. loss of bladder and bowel functions
6. loss of movement and sensation in the limbs
7. loss of consciousness

If the damage to the brain is extensive, patients may die within a few days to a few weeks.

LONG-TERM EFFECTS OF PENETRATING TBI

The long-term effects of penetrating TBI among survivors include impairment of the following neurological functions:

1. cognitive (attention and memory)
2. motor (extreme weakness, poor coordination and balance)
3. sensation (hearing, vision, impaired perception, and touch)
4. emotion (depression, anxiety, aggression, impulse control, and personality changes)
5. post-traumatic stress disorder (PTSD)

The survivors of penetrating TBI may face long-term serious disabilities that can cause a very poor quality of life. These disabilities may include brain damage and the development of post-traumatic stress disorder (PTSD). In order to determine the amount of damage done to the brain, a scoring system is used. Some of them are discussed below.

TBI SCORING SYSTEMS

The Glasgow Coma Score (GCS) is one of the most commonly used scoring systems; it is designed to measure the severity level of a brain injury. Individuals with GCS scores of 3–8 are classified as having a severe TBI; those with scores of 9–12 are classified as having a moderate TBI; and those with scores of 13–15 are classified as having a mild TBI. Other classification systems include the Abbreviated Injury Scale (AIS), the Revised Trauma Score, and the Injury Severity Score. These classifications are useful in the clinical management of TBI, and the scores of one or more of the above classifications are useful in predicting clinical outcomes.

BRAIN DAMAGE IN PATIENTS
WITH PENETRATING TBI

Brain damage after penetrating TBI is very complex, depending upon the type and velocity of the inducing agents, the area and the size of the affected brain tissue, and the amount of brain tissue lost. Generally, swelling, edema, hematoma, hemorrhage, contusion, focal cerebral vasospasm, increased blood-brain barrier (BBB) permeability, and diffuse axonal injury are commonly observed immediately after injury (Hicks et al. 2010).

It has been reported that penetrating ballisticlike injury and hemorrhagic shock can cause persistent damage of cerebral blood flow and a reduced supply of oxygen to the brain, which also contributes to the progression of brain damage by compromising neurological recovery (Leung et al. 2013).

RISK OF DEVELOPING
POST-TRAUMATIC STRESS DISORDER (PTSD)
AMONG SURVIVORS OF MILD TBI

Epidemiologic studies (survey types of studies) on the relationship between TBI and PTSD among U.S. soldiers returning from Iraq and Afghanistan reported that among 2,525 soldiers, 4.9 percent reported injury with loss of consciousness, 10.3 percent reported injuries with altered mental status, and 17.2 percent reported other injuries during deployment. Among those who reported loss of consciousness, the incidence of PTSD was about 43.9 percent. Among those reporting altered mental status, it was 27.3 percent. For those reporting other injuries, the incidence of PTSD was 16.2 percent.

In contrast, in those soldiers reporting no injury in combat, the incidence of PTSD was only 9.1 percent (Schneiderman, Braver, and Kang 2008). It was proposed that the strong association between mild TBI and PTSD may be due to life-threatening combat experiences; in some cases, it could reflect neurological deficits as well as traumatic stress. Female soldiers had a higher incidence of PTSD than did male soldiers.

INCIDENCE AND PREVELANCE
OF PENETRATING TBI

American troops in combat are at a high risk of sustaining penetrating TBI given that approximately 65 percent of soldiers are injured by explosive devices. Because of excellent trauma care in the battlefield, the number of survivors has increased, resulting in higher number of soldiers with TBI who face a long rehabilitative process and who suffer from various neurological disorders.

The Center for Disease Control and Prevention (CDC) estimates that about 1.7 million people sustain TBI (concussion and penetrating forms) each year. TBI accounts for about 30.5 percent of all injury-related deaths and for substantial cases of permanent disability. The CDC has estimated that at least 5.3 million Americans who suffer from TBI have a long-term or lifelong need for assistance in performing the activities of daily living.

COSTS OF TBI

The costs per year per person with mild TBI is about $32,000; moderate to severe TBI is approximately $268,000 to more than $408,000. In 2010, the direct medical and indirect costs (such as lost productivity) were estimated to be $76.5 billion.

BIOCHEMICAL DEFECTS THAT CONTRIBUTE TO THE PROGRESSION OF DAMAGE IN SEVERE TBI

Both animal and human studies show that severe TBI causes a significant loss of cortical tissue at the site of injury (primary damage); this invariably is followed by secondary damage. This secondary damage may take the form of abnormal biochemical defects such as increased oxidative damage, mitochondrial dysfunction, and the release of predominantly pro-inflammatory cytokines and glutamate, all of which may lead to neurological dysfunction and neuronal death. Therefore, attenuation of these biochemical defects in TBI patients may help to reduce the progression of damage. When combined with standard therapy, this would improve the management of severe TBI more than would be produced by standard therapy alone.

Evidence of Increased
Oxidative Stress in Penetrating TBI

Both animal and human studies suggest that increased oxidative stress plays an important role in the progression of injury after penetrating TBI. Some studies are described here.

In Animal Studies

Increased oxidative stress due to the production of excessive amounts of free radicals derived from oxygen and nitrogen occurs after penetrating TBI (Bayir, Kochanek, and Kagan 2006; Rael et al. 2009; Shao et al. 2006).

Increased production of superoxide radicals has been demonstrated in mice models of TBI (Mikawa et al. 1996).

In a rat model of TBI, the extent of oxidative damage appeared to be directly proportional to the severity of the TBI (Petronilho et al. 2009).

In rats, the total antioxidant reserves of ascorbate, glutathione, and sulfhydryl proteins were reduced after a TBI (Singh, Sullivan, and Hall 2007).

It has been shown that TBI increased the production of nitric oxide (NO), which can be oxidized to form another form of free radical, peroxynitrite. This form of free radical also damages mitochondria, resulting in reduced energy production (Huttemann et al. 2008).

TBI also increased inducible nitric oxide synthase (iNOS) activity. This increases the production of NO, which can be oxidized to form peroxynitrite. Peroxynitrite contributes to neurological deficits but not to cerebral edema (Louin et al. 2006).

In a rat model of traumatic injury (unilateral moderate cortical contusion), increased oxidative damage occurred as early as three hours following TBI. This adversely affected synaptic function and the plasticity of hippocampal neurons, and thereby enhanced cognitive dysfunction (Ansari, Roberts, and Scheff 2008).

In another model of TBI (fluid percussion brain injury in rats), it was observed that protein carbonylation (oxidation of protein) and thiobarbituric acid-reactive substance (TBARS) levels increased in the cortex 1 and 3 months following the injury. These changes in markers of oxidative damage may account for the cognitive dysfunction observed following TBI (Lima et al. 2008).

The levels of antioxidant enzymes Mn-SOD (manganese-dependent superoxide dismutase) and glutathione reductase decreased more in older rats than in the younger ones following TBI. The levels of markers of oxidative damage such as products of lipid peroxidation (acrolein and 4-hydroxynonenal) increased more in older rats than in younger rats (Shao et al. 2006).

In rats, there appears to be a close relationship between the degree of oxidative stress and the severity of brain damage following TBI, as evidenced by the highest value of malondialdehyde (MDA) and the lowest value of ascorbate (Tavazzi et al. 2005).

It has been found that activation of the Nrf2/ARE pathway, which increases the levels of antioxidant enzymes, is enhanced during early brain damage after inducing subarachnoid hemorrhage in rats (Chen et al. 2011). Since transient increased oxidative stress is required for the activation of the Nrf2/ARE pathway, it can be concluded that increased oxidative stress occurred as an early biochemical defect that may contribute to the progression of damage after TBI.

In Human Studies

A few human studies also confirm the role of oxidative stress in the progression of TBI. F2- isoprostane is a marker of lipid peroxidation, and neuron-specific enolase (NSE) is considered a marker of neuronal damage. The levels of F2-isoprostane and NSE increased in cerebral spinal fluid (CSF) samples following TBI in children and infants (Varma et al. 2003).

Both the levels of ascorbate and glutathione also decreased in the

CSF of children and infants following TBI (Bayir et al. 2002).

Metabolic function of the brain in children with penetrating TBI is impaired. Although cerebral blood flow is variable after severe TBI in children, a low oxygen metabolic index and hypoperfusion (reduced blood supply to the brain) were observed (Ragan et al. 2013).

A clinical study showed that the level of 3-nitrotyrosine increased in the CSF of patients with TBI (Darwish, Amiridze, and Aarabi 2007).

Another clinical study reported that increased levels of cytochrome C and activated caspase-9 were detected in the CSF of adult patients with severe TBI (Darwish and Amiridze 2010). Increased levels of cytochrome C and activated caspase-9 play a significant role in causing neuronal death.

In a clinical study on 106 healthy individuals and 106 patients with severe TBI (GCS score of 1–3), it was demonstrated that the plasma levels of 8-iso-prostaglandin F2alpha, a marker of oxidative damage in vivo, were higher in patients with severe TBI than in healthy individuals (Yu et al. 2013).

Another clinical study has shown a close relationship between oxidative stress and glutamate-induced damage following severe TBI in humans (Clausen et al. 2012).

A clinical study on 30 severe TBI patients (with a GCS score of 8 or less), 20 patients with mild TBI and 36 age-sex-matched healthy individuals showed that the levels of erythrocyte thiobarbituric acid substances (TBARS) were significantly higher, and levels of glutathione were lower, in patients with mild and severe TBI compared to those of healthy individuals. (Nayak et al. 2008).

In another clinical study, it was demonstrated that plasma levels of TBARS and protein oxidation (carbonyl) increased significantly in the first 70 hours after severe TBI (Hohl et al. 2012).

It has been reported that the levels of beta-amyloid fragments (generated from the cleavage of amyloid precursor protein) increased in the cerebral spinal fluid of patients after severe TBI (Emmerling et al. 2000).

These amyloid fragments have been implicated in causing neuronal damage via increased production of free radicals in patients with Alzheimer's disease. One of the mechanisms of damage caused by beta-amyloid fragments involves increased oxidative stress (Pappolla et al. 1998; Butterfield 2002).

The studies discussed above suggest that agents that can decrease oxidative stress could be useful in prevention and in reducing the progression of damage after severe TBI in humans. This issue will be discussed in detail in chapter 8.

Oxidative Stress and Mitochondrial Dysfunction in Penetrating TBI

Most free radicals are produced in the mitochondria. Mitochondria are easily damaged by free radicals. Both animal and human studies suggest that mitochondrial dysfunction plays an important role in the progression of injury after severe TBI. A few studies are described here.

In Animal Studies

Increased oxidative stress contributes to the mitochondrial dysfunction that plays an important role in causing cognitive impairment and eventually neuronal death following TBI (Robertson et al. 2009; Mazzeo et al. 2009).

A significant loss of brain tissue at the site of damage occurs immediately after severe TBI; this is referred to as primary damage. After that, secondary damage, which includes mitochondrial dysfunction, occurs. This leads to various neurological disorders. In a rat model of TBI, several mitochondrial proteins involved in producing energy were damaged by free radicals causing mitochondrial dysfunction, which eventually leads to neuronal death in the brain (Opii et al. 2007).

In addition, it was found that the activity of mitochondrial enzyme pyruvate dehydrogenase (PDH) decreased, acid-based balances were disrupted, and levels of oxidative stress increased in the rats' blood. The decrease in blood levels of PDH was associated with increased gliosis (increased proliferation of glia cells, an indication of the presence of inflammation in the brain) (Sharma et al. 2009). These biochemical changes contribute to the severity of brain injury.

Generally, oxidative stress-induced mitochondrial dysfunction in a rat model of TBI is observed 1 to 3 hours after the TBI, suggesting the importance of an early intervention to reduce the resultant oxidative stress (Gilmer et al. 2009).

In a mouse model of TBI, it was observed that mitochondrial damage in the cortex included swelling, disruption of membranous structures, and reduction of the calcium-buffering capacity, and an elevation of oxidation of protein and lipids. The levels of 3-nitrotyrosine, a marker of nitrosylative damage, were elevated as early as 30 minutes after injury (Singh et al. 2006).

N-methyl-4-isoleucine-cyclosporin (NIM811), a nonimmuno-suppressive cyclosporine A analog, inhibits the mitochondrial permeability transition pore. Supplementation with NIM811 improved mitochondrial function and cognitive function and reduced oxidative damage in a severe unilateral controlled cortical impact rat model of TBI (Readnower et al. 2011).

Mitochondrial dysfunction can further increase oxidative damage, loss of respiratory functions, and diminished ability to buffer cytosolic calcium, all of which can cause neuronal death in the brain. In the mouse model, it was demonstrated that supplementation with U-83836E, a potent inhibitor of lipid peroxyl radicals, reduced both oxidative and nitrosylative damage in the neurons and the mitochondria after severe TBI (Mustafa et al. 2010)

In Human Studies

It has been reported that mitochondrial DNA polymorphism (more than one variant of a gene) was associated with mitochondrial dysfunction and behavioral abnormalities after severe TBI (Conley et al. 2013). Mitochondrial dysfunction increases the production of free radicals. There is a direct link between energy metabolism and n-acetylaspartate.

In a clinical study of 14 patients (6 patients with diffuse brain injury and 8 with focal brain lesions), it was observed that reduction in the brain levels of n-acetylaspartate in the absence of ischemic insult reflected mitochondrial dysfunction (Aygok et al. 2008).

It has been proposed that reduction in extracellular levels of n-acetylaspartate can be used as a potential marker of mitochondrial dysfunction in humans after TBI (Belli et al. 2006). The role of mitochondrial dysfunction in the progression of damage following TBI is further supported by the fact that, in rats, treatment with mitochondrial uncouplers, 2,4-dinitrophenol (2,4-DNP) and p-trifluoromethoxyphenylhydrazone (FCCP), significantly reduced the loss of brain neurons and improved behavioral functions following TBI (Pandya et al. 2007).

The studies discussed above suggest that agents that can reduce oxidative stress and reduce mitochondrial dysfunction could be useful in reducing the progression of damage after severe TBI in humans. This issue will be discussed in detail in chapter 8.

Evidence of Increased Inflammation in Severe TBI

Both animal and human studies suggest that increased inflammation plays an important role in the progression of injury after severe TBI. A few studies are described here.

In Animal Studies

The levels of inflammation markers, such as iNOS (inducible nitric oxide synthase) and cyclooxygenase 2 (COX-2) activities, and markers of oxidative damage, such as reduced levels of glutathione, 3-nitrotyrosine, and 4-hydroxynonenal, increased after severe TBI in an animal model. Treatment with fenofibrate reduced the levels of these markers (Chen et al. 2007).

In rats, the levels of pro-inflammatory cytokines, and tumor necrosis factor-alpha (TNF-alpha) increased after TBI.

The delayed elevation of soluble tumor necrosis factor receptors p75 and p55 was observed in the cerebral spinal fluid (CSF) and plasma after TBI (Maier et al. 2006).

The levels of TNF-alpha and Fas are elevated after TBI. Using TNF-alpha and Fas deficient transgenic mice (TNF-alpha/Fas-/-), it was demonstrated that the motor performance and spatial memory acquisition were improved in these transgenic mice subjected to TBI compared to wild type mice subjected to TBI. The results suggested that TNF-alpha and Fas play an important role in TBI-induced neurological dysfunction. This was further supported by the fact that in immature normal mice subjected to TBI, genetic inhibition of TNF-alpha and Fas reduced neuronal loss and improved memory function in adulthood (Bermpohl et al. 2007).

Nuclear factor erythroid-2-related factor 2 (Nrf2) is an important transcriptional factor that provides protection against toxic products of inflammation. Using a transgenic mice deficient in Nrf2 (-/-), it was demonstrated that activation of NF-kappaB, the levels of pro-inflammatory cytokines, TNF-alpha, IL-1beta and IL-6, and expression of intracellular adhesion molecule 1 (ICAN-1) were higher in the brain compared to the wild type Nrf2 (+/+) mice following TBI (moderate to severe weight-drop impact head injury) (Jin et al. 2008; Jin et al. 2009).

The role of pro-inflammatory cytokines in the progression of damage after TBI is further supported by the fact that inhibitors of these cytokines reduced neuronal loss and cognitive dysfunction in animal models of TBI. For example, it was shown that the following agents protected the brain by reducing neuronal loss and neurological deficits:

- IL-1 beta neutralizing antibody (IgG2a/k) (Clausen et al. 2009);
- dexanabinol (HU-211), an inhibitor of TNF-alpha antioxidants (Shohami et al. 1997);
- an inhibitor of inflammation (Trembovler et al. 1999);
- Minozac (Mzc), an inhibitor of glial activation and pro-inflammatory cytokines (Lloyd et al. 2008);
- a synthetic analogue of tripeptide Glypromate (NNZ-2566) (Wei et al. 2009);
- an inhibitor of activation of astrocytes;
- and simvastatin, a cholesterol lowering drug (Wu et al. 2009).

In Human Studies

A review of the role of inflammation in penetrating TBI has revealed that a strong inflammatory response occurs immediately after injury. Inflammatory response activates resident glia cells, microglia and astrocytes, which secrete pro-inflammatory cytokines (IL-1, IL-6, and TNF-alpha) and anti-inflammatory cytokines (IL-4, IL-10, and TGF-beta), and chemokines (Woodcock and Morganti-Kossmann 2013).

Examination of the 21 autopsied brain samples of patients with severe TBI showed that the levels of pro-inflammatory cytokines were elevated, whereas the levels of anti-inflammatory cytokines did not change (Frugier et al. 2010).

This is in contrast to the acute phase of TBI when both pro- and anti-inflammatory cytokines are released (Woodcock and Morganti-Kossmann 2013).

It has been demonstrated that activated microglia persists as long as 17 years after injury (Ramlackhansingh et al. 2011). These studies are very important for dose-schedule of anti-inflammatory agents after TBI. If an inhibitor of inflammation is administered immediately after injury, the release of both anti- and pro-inflammatory cytokines may be reduced. The decreased levels of anti-inflammatory cytokines may interfere with the repair of brain injury after TBI.

Diffuse Axonal Injury

Diffuse axonal injury after TBI is the leading cause of lasting vegetative state and death of patients. A clinical study of 159 patients with severe TBI who survived the acute phase of TBI showed that about 72 percent of the patients had diffused axonal injury (Skandsen et al. 2010).

A review has shown that increased levels of pro-inflammatory cytokines play an important role in the development and progression of diffuse axonal injury (Lin and Wen 2013).

After TBI, activated microglia in the brain generate excessive amounts of pro-inflammatory cytokines, prostaglandins, reactive oxygen species (ROS), complement proteins, and adhesion molecules that are highly toxic to neurons (Goodman et al. 2008; Hutchinson et al. 2007; Hein and O'Banion 2009).

Evidence of inflammation is also found by the infiltration and accumulation of polymorphonuclear leukocytes. Pro-inflammatory cytokines increased the expression of iNOS (inducible nitric oxide synthase), which can produce excessive amounts of NO (nitric oxide) that may in turn become oxidized to form peroxynitrite, which contributes to the progression of TBI (Potts et al. 2006; Hall et al. 2004).

An inhibitor of iNOS protected neurons from damage produced by peroxynitrite (Gahm et al. 2006). The pro-inflammatory cytokine interleukin-6 (IL-6) is elevated in patients with severe TBI. A significant relationship exists between the severity of TBI and the levels of IL-6 in the brain (Minambres 2003).

Cytokines in Infants and Children with TBI

Severe TBI in 36 infants and children increased the levels of pro-inflammatory cytokines (IL-1beta, IL-6, and IL-12p70) and anti-inflammatory cytokines (IL-10) and chemokines (IL-8 and MIP-1 alpha), compared to those who did not sustain TBI. Moderate hypothermia did not decrease the levels of cytokines in children with TBI (Buttram et al. 2007).

Evidence of Increased Glutamate Release in Severe TBI

Both animal and human studies suggest that increased levels of extracellular glutamate plays an important role in the progression of injury after severe TBI. A few studies are described here.

In Animal Studies

The levels of extracellular glutamate and aspartate increased in the brain regions of animals following TBI (Gopinath et al. 2000).

In a rat model of TBI, it was shown that the levels of 2 high-affinity sodium-dependent glial transporters, glutamate transporter 1(GLT-1) and glutamate-aspartame transporter (GLAST), decreased following TBI (Rao et al. 1998; Yi and Hazell 2006). Glutamate transporter GLT-1 is primarily responsible for clearing extracellular glutamate, therefore, decreased levels of GLT-1 may contribute to increased levels of extracellular glutamate in the brain. Thus, increased levels of GLT-1 may protect neurons from TBI-induced damage by reducing the extracellular levels of glutamate.

This is supported by the observation that administration of ceftriaxone, which increases the expression of GLT-1, reversed TBI-induced elevation of glia fibrillary acid protein (GFAP) and seizures in a rat model of TBI (Goodrich et al. 2013).

It has been reported that an increase in glia-regulated release of extracellular glutamate contributes to the progression of damage in the striatum of rats 2 days after diffuse brain injury (Hinzman et al. 2012).

It has been demonstrated that increase in the levels of extracellular glutamate occurs due to excessive release of glutamate from the neurons (Hascup et al. 2010). Thus, both neurons and glia contribute to the increased levels of extracellular glutamate after TBI.

In a rat model of TBI, hypothermia treatment, which provides neuroprotection, reduced the levels of hydroxyl radicals and glutamate release (Globus et al. 1995).

Administration of N-methyl-D-aspartame, a (NMDA) antagonist, significantly reduced glutamate release, and improved motor function and reduced cognitive dysfunction following TBI in animal models (Panter and Faden 1992).

It has been demonstrated that injection of premarin, a conjugated estrogen commonly used as hormone replacement therapy in postmenopausal women, decreased blood glutamate levels in a rat model of TBI (Zlotnik et al. 2012).

The extracellular levels of glutamate and adenosine increase rapidly after TBI, however, the relationship between them in the progression of injury is not well understood. Normally, adenosine a (2A) receptor (A2AR) exerts protective effects on the brain, but it can contribute to degeneration of nerve cells, depending upon the levels of glutamate. It has been demonstrated that a high concentration of glutamate switched the effect of activated A2AR from anti-inflammatory to proinflammatory in microglia cells in culture and in a mouse model of TBI (Dai et al. 2010).

In Human Studies

Glutamate plays a significant role in the progression of injury following severe TBI. Excessive amounts of glutamate in the extracellular space of the brain may lead to uncontrolled shifts of sodium, potassium, and calcium, which may cause swelling, edema, and eventually cell death.

In addition, increased synaptic release of glutamate occurs at the site of injury (Yi and Hazell 2006).

In a clinical study of 80 patients with severe head injury, it was observed that the levels of glutamate increased, which may enhance neuronal damage in these patients (Bullock et al. 1998).

In patients with focal and diffuse brain injury, the levels of glutamate were elevated in both the cerebrospinal fluid and extracellular space of the brain following TBI (Yamamoto et al. 1999).

In another clinical study, it was found that patients who died of their head injury had higher levels of dialysate glutamate and aspartate compared to those who recovered from injury. The highest levels of glutamate and aspartate were present in patients with gunshot wounds, followed by those who had mass lesions.

A clinical study of 85 severely head-injured patients showed that excessive amounts of glutamate and aspartate were released. Patients with contusions were found to have the highest level of glutamate and aspartate (Koura et al. 1998).

In a clinical study of 28 severely brain-injured patients, the levels of glutamate and taurine in the ventricular cerebrospinal fluid (CSF) were elevated. The simultaneous release of taurine, which has inhibitory and anti-excitotoxic functions, with glutamate, suggests that the injured brain is attempting to counteract the action of glutamate (Stover et al. 1999).

Similar results were obtained in a rat model of TBI (Stover and Unterberg 2000).

A clinical study of 165 patients with severe TBI showed that the increased levels of glutamate measured by microdialysis were correlated with higher mortality and poor functional outcomes (Chamoun et al. 2010).

The concentration of glutamate and glycerol in microdialysate from older patients with severe TBI were higher compared to younger patients (Mellergard, Sjogren, and Hillman 2012). This suggested that increased concentrations of glycerol and glutamate would indicate more extensive damage in older patients.

A clinical study of 223 individuals with severe TBI showed that higher concentrations of glutamate, glucose, lactate/pyruvate ratio, intracranial pressure, cerebral cerebrovascular pressure, and age were predictors of increased mortality (Timofeev et al. 2011).

In a clinical study of 27 children with severe TBI and 21 children without TBI or meningitis, it was observed that the levels of adenosine and glutamate were elevated in the ventricular CSF following TBI. The release of adenosine following TBI may reflect an attempt by adenosine to protect nerve cells from glutamate-induced toxicity (Robertson et al. 2001).

CONCLUDING REMARKS

Damage to the brain after penetrating TBI occurs in three phases. The first phase involves loss of brain tissue that cannot be restored. The second phase of TBI occurs soon after injury and continues for days to weeks; intervention with appropriate agents can slow down the progression of damage. The third phase of severe TBI appears as late effects that may include cognitive dysfunction, PTSD, and other behavioral abnormalities.

Some individuals who have suffered a penetrating TBI may die within a few days or weeks. The survivors of penetrating TBI may face long-term serious disabilities that can cause a very poor quality of life. These disabilities may include the development of post-traumatic stress disorder (PTSD). In general, the rate of recovery for anyone who has undergone a severe TBI is typically unique to the individual as it depends upon a variety of factors. And although many individuals with severe penetrating TBI may undergo a long rehabilitation process, even mild penetrating TBI can have devastating effects on the afflicted individual, their families, and friends.

Soldiers may be the group at the highest risk of developing severe TBI, given that 65 percent of combat personnel are injured by IEDs. In terms of the civilian population, approximately 1.7 million people suffer from TBI on an annual basis.

The animal and human studies presented in this chapter imply that oxidative stress and inflammation are largely responsible for the progression of damage following a penetrating TBI. The inclusion of recommended micronutrients as well as modifications in the diet and lifestyle may prove useful in reducing this progression of damage following penetrating TBI. We will explore this topic more extensively in the following chapter.

8 Treating and Managing Penetrating TBI with Vitamins and Antioxidants

Although there has been significant improvement in the management of penetrating TBI, treatment strategies for patients with this condition remain unsatisfactory. There is no effective strategy to reduce the risk of dementia and other forms of mental disorders associated with it, and the incidence of morbidity following penetrating TBI continues to be high. Despite measures such as standardized treatment guidelines, several clinical studies aimed at identifying therapeutic agents, and improved understanding of the mechanisms of cellular damage, this remains the case. In order to develop a rational strategy for reducing the progression of damage inflicted by a penetrating TBI, it's important to identify major biological events that play a crucial role in the progression of this type of injury.

In attempting to achieve that goal, this chapter discusses some antioxidant studies of animals and humans undertaken following severe TBI. This chapter also presents scientific rationale and evidence in support of our primary recommendation: Daily supplementation with a preparation of micronutrients containing dietary and endogenous antioxidants and certain polyphenolic compounds, in combination with standard care, may reduce the progressive damage and improve the acute and long-term management of penetrating TBI. This combination of therapies may reduce the extent of brain damage during the first and second phases of injury, perhaps even more effectively than standard care alone.

THE EFFECT OF A SINGLE ANTIOXIDANT IN STUDIES OF PENETRATING TBI

In Animal Studies

Resveratrol

Resveratrol, a polyphenolic compound isolated from grape seeds, administered immediately after TBI reduced oxidative damage and neuronal loss in rat brains (Ates et al. 2007; Sonmez et al. 2007).

Alpha-lipoic Acid and N-acetylcysteine

Treatment with alpha-lipoic acid reduced markers of pro-inflammatory cytokines and oxidative stress, and improved survival of neurons in the brain, preserved blood-brain-barrier (BBB) permeability, and reduced edema following TBI in animals (Toklu et al. 2009). Administration of n-acetylcysteine (NAC) provided neuroprotection (reduction in brain edema and BBB permeability) by reducing markers of pro-inflammatory cytokines and adhesion molecules in an animal model of TBI (Chen et al. 2008).

The early rise in complex I and complex II proteins of mitochondria that regulate excitatory neurotransmitter release following TBI was blocked by n-acetylcysteine (NAC) (Yi et al. 2006).

In addition, TBI-induced elevation of heme oxygenase-1 (HO-1) levels in glial cells as well as neurons, and loss of neurons from the brain was markedly reduced by NAC treatment in an animal model of TBI (Yi and Hazell 2005).

Vitamin E and Curcumin

Dietary supplementation with vitamin E or curcumin protected the brain against mild TBI-induced damage by reducing the above biochemical changes involved in synaptic plasticity and cognitive function in rats (Wu, Ying, and Gomez-Pinilla 2006).

Omega-3 Fatty Acids

It has been reported that dietary supplementation with omega-3 fatty acids in an animal model of TBI (mild fluid-percussion injury) protected against TBI-induced reduced synaptic plasticity and cognitive impairment (Wu, Ying, and Gomez-Pinilla 2011).

In contrast, supplementation with a saturated fat diet (Wu et al. 2003) or caffeine (Al Moutaery et al. 2003) aggravated TBI-induced injury in animals.

Antioxidant Enzymes

Superoxide dismutase improved TBI-induced mitochondrial dysfunction in transgenic mice over-expressing CuZn SOD or Mn SOD (Xiong et al. 2005).

In transgenic mice over-expressing glutathione peroxidase (GPxTg), it was observed that markers of oxidative stress including nitrotyrosine were reduced and spatial memory improved compared to wild type animals following TBI (Tsuru-Aoyagi et al. 2009).

Melatonin

Melatonin, a pineal hormone necessary for sleep, exhibited antioxidant activity and protected against TBI-induced damage by attenuating the activation of NF-kappaB and AP-1 (Beni et al. 2004).

S-nitrosoglutathione (GSNO)

S-nitrosoglutathione (GSNO), a modulator of nitric oxide, plays an important role in maintaining a balance between oxidants and antioxidants in the body. Administration of GSNO after severe TBI reduced blood-brain barrier disruption, infiltration/activation of macrophages, and reduced expression of ICAM-1, MMP- and iNOS. This treatment also reduced neuronal cell loss and myelin loss in rats (Khan et al. 2009).

In Human Studies

Edaravone

In humans, Edaravone, an FDA approved drug, reduced oxidative damage by neutralizing free radicals after TBI (Dohi et al. 2006).

PROPOSED PREVENTION STRATEGIES IN PENETRATING TBI

Primary Prevention of Penetrating TBI
Given the sudden and typically unexpected nature of a traumatic brain injury, primary prevention strategies for penetrating TBI cannot be developed.

Secondary Prevention of Severe TBI
The purpose of secondary prevention is to slow the progression of severe TBI in order to reduce the risk of developing edema, increased cerebral vascular permeability, and neuronal death during the acute phase of injury. The purpose of secondary prevention is also to reduce the risk of developing late adverse health effects, such as cognitive dysfunction, PTSD, and behavior abnormalities among those who survive severe TBI. During the acute phase of severe TBI, excessive amounts of free radicals and inflammation, which play an important role in the progression of acute injury, are produced.

The formulation of micronutrients (table 8.1) is recommended for secondary prevention. However, the micronutrients should be administered 24–48 hours after severe TBI. This is due to the fact that both pro- and anti-inflammatory cytokines are released during the acute phase of injury. Anti-inflammatory cytokines are necessary for the healing processes. Any inhibition of inflammation by micronutrients soon after severe TBI occurs may impair the potential repair processes by reducing anti-inflammatory cytokines. Therefore, supplementation with a preparation of micronutrients containing dietary and endogenous antioxidants, polyphenolic compounds (resveratrol and curcumin) and omega-3 fatty acids may be one of the rational choices for secondary prevention of penetrating TBI. This is due to the fact that innumerable amounts of free radicals and toxic products of inflammation occur soon after injury and these supplemented micronutrients are capable of optimally reducing oxidative stress and inflammation.

A formulation for the secondary prevention of penetrating TBI for adults is provided in table 8.1 on page 122.

Standard Therapy in Secondary Prevention of Severe TBI

Severe TBI is extremely difficult to treat because of the inherent complexity of the brain's structures and functions as well as extreme variations in patterns of injury. Standard therapy, however, has markedly improved the management of severe TBI and has improved the survival rate of those suffering from it. Approximately half of severely brain-injured patients will need surgery to remove or repair hematomas (rupture of blood vessels) or contusions (bruised brain tissue) (National Institute of Neurological Disorders and Stroke, 2009).

Initial treatment of standard therapy focuses on preventing secondary injury following TBI. This includes ensuring a proper oxygen supply to the brain and the rest of the body, maintaining adequate blood flow, and controlling blood pressure. Hypothermia (reducing the body's temperature to 32–34°C) has been used in the management of TBI.

TABLE 8.1. FORMULATION OF A MICRONUTRIENT PREPARATION FOR SECONDARY PREVENTION OF PENETRATING TRAUMATIC BRAIN INJURY (TBI) IN ADULTS*

Vitamin A (as palmitate)	3,000
Vitamin C (as calcium ascorbate)	1,000 mg
Natural Vitamin E	400 IU (as d-alpha-tocpheryl succinate 250 IU) (as d-alpha-tocopheryl acetate 150 IU)
Vitamin D (as cholocalciferol)	1,000 IU
Vitamin B_1 (thiamine mononitrate)	10 mg
Vitamin B_2 (riboflavin)	4 mg
Nicotinamide (as nicotinamide ascorbate)	100 mg
Vitamin B_6 (as pyrodioxine HCl)	4 mg
Folate (folic acid)	800 mcg
Vitamin B_{12} (as cyanocobalamin)	100 mcg
Biotin	150 mcg
Pantothenic acid (as d-calcium pantothenate)	15 mg
Zinc (as zinc glycinate)	5 mg
Selenium (as selenomethionine)	100 mcg
Coenzyme Q10	proprietary amount[†]
N-acetylcysteine	proprietary amount
R-alpha-lipoic acid	proprietary amount
Natural mixed carotenoids	proprietary amount
Curcumin	proprietary amount
Resveratrol	proprietary amount
Omega-3 fatty acids	proprietary amount

*Total capsules perday can be taken orally, half in the morning and half in the evening.
[†]Total amounts of antioxidants and herbal products come to 1,585 mg

In a clinical study, it was demonstrated that hypothermia attenuated the levels of markers of oxidative stress in infants and children following severe TBI (Bayir et al. 2009).

The effect of hypothermia was analyzed in 12 studies with 1,327 patients in which 8 studies cooled patients according to a long-term strategy for a period of about 3 to 5 days, and 4 studies cooled patients according to short-term strategy for a period of about 1.5 to 2.5 days. The results revealed that when patients were cooled for a short period of time, neither mortality rates nor neurological outcomes were improved. However, when the patients were cooled for a longer period of time, mortality was reduced and neurological outcomes were improved (Fox et al. 2010). The optimal results were obtained when the patients were cooled for at least 72 hours and/or until intracranial pressure was normalized for at least 24 hours.

In children with penetrating TBI, the CSF levels of alpha-synuclein were elevated in patients with TBI more than in control subjects, however, the CSF levels of alpha-synuclein decreased after hypothermia treatment (Su et al. 2010).

Medications to reduce secondary damage to the brain immediately after injury may include the following:

1. Diuretics (to reduce pressure in the brain by eliminating fluid through the urine)
2. Anti-seizure drugs administered during the first week post-injury (to avoid additional damage to the brain that might be caused by seizures)
3. Coma-inducing drugs (brains in this state use less oxygen for survival and function; this procedure is particularly helpful if the blood vessels are unable to supply sufficient nutrients and oxygen to the brain)
   a. emergency surgery may be needed to remove blood clots, repair skull fractures, and open a window in the skull to

relieve pressure inside the brain by draining accumulated fluid, and;

b. rehabilitation therapy that includes an individually tailored treatment program, such as physical therapy, occupational therapy, speech/language therapy, psychological/psychiatric therapy, and social support

Based on the studies on animal models of TBI, several potentially therapeutic agents have been identified. They include erythropoietin (Grasso et al. 2007; Xiong, Chopp, and Lee 2009); antibodies of serotonin receptors (Sharma et al. 2007); histone deacetylase inhibitors (Zhang et al. 2008; Dash et al. 2010); protease inhibitors (Foley, Kast, and Altschuler 2009); fenofibrate, a peroxisomes proliferators-activated receptor alpha agonist (Chen et al. 2007); meloxicam, a COX-2 inhibitor (Hakan et al. 2009); and interferon-gamma. (Chen et al. 2009). These drugs have not been approved by the FDA for the treatment of human penetrating TBI.

Recommended Micronutrients in Combination with Standard Therapy in Secondary Prevention of Severe TBI

Individuals who sustain penetrating TBI provide an excellent opportunity to study the efficacy of a multiple micronutrient preparation, in combination with standard therapy, to reduce secondary damage during the acute and chronic phase of injury. These patients require immediate emergency care in the hospital to receive standard therapy in order to stabilize their conditions.

A separate preparation of micronutrients, in combination with standard therapy, is recommended during the acute phase of injury (see table 8.2 on page 126). It should be pointed out that oral supplementation with a preparation of micronutrient should be started 24 hours after injury, not immediately after injury. This is due to the fact that both anti- and pro-inflammatory cytokines are released immediately after injury. Anti-inflammatory cytokines help to repair cellular damage. Supplementation with a preparation of micronutrient immediately after injury may reduce both pro-inflammatory and anti-inflammatory cytokines. Inhibition of anti-inflammatory cytokines release may interfere with the repair processes in the brain.

The above-listed micronutrients should be administered orally twice a day in powder form mixed with liquid, half in the morning and half in the evening, 24–48 hours after injury. This treatment with a preparation of micronutrients should be continued for four to six weeks, after which the formulation for secondary prevention (table 8.1) should be adopted for the entire lifespan in order to reduce the late adverse health effects of penetrating TBI.

Diet and Lifestyle Recommendations for Penetrating TBI

In addition to supplementation with multiple micronutrients, a balanced diet is very necessary to reduce the risk of long-term adverse effects on brain functions, as well as to improve the efficacy of standard therapy in the management of acute and long-term management of penetrating TBI. I recommend a balanced low-fat diet containing plenty of fruits and vegetables. Lifestyle recommendations include daily moderate exercise, reduced stress, no tobacco smoking, and a reduced intake of caffeine. A diet high in saturated fat diet (Wu et al. 2003) and caffeine (Al Moutaery et al. 2003) appears to increase the progression of damage following TBI in animal models.

TABLE 8.2. FORMULATION OF A MICRONUTRIENT PREPARATION FOR ADULTS WHO HAVE SUSTAINED SEVERE TRAUMATIC BRAIN INJURY (TBI)*

Vitamin A (as palmitate)	5,000 IU
Vitamin C (as calcium ascorbate)	2,000 mg
Vitamin E	400 IU (as d-alpha-tocpheryl succinate 200 IU) (as d-alpha-tocopheryl acetate 200 IU)
Vitamin D (as cholocalciferol)	1,000 IU
Vitamin B_1 (thiamine mononitrate)	10 mg
Vitamin B_2 (riboflavin)	5mg
Nicotinamide (as nicotinamide ascorbate)	150 mg
Vitamin B_6 (as pyrodioxine HCl)	4 mg
Folate (folic acid)	400 mcg
Vitamin B_{12} (as methyl cobalamin)	150 mcg
Biotin	200 mcg
Pantothenic acid (as d-calcium pantothenate)	10 mg
Zinc (as zinc glycinate)	15 mg
Selenium (as selenomethionine)	200 mcg
Chromium (as chromium picolinate)	50 mcg
Coenzyme Q10	proprietary amount[†]
N-acetylcysteine	proprietary amount
Alpha-lipoic acid	proprietary amount
Natural mixed carotenoids	proprietary amount
Curcumin	proprietary amount
Resveratrol	proprietary amount
Omega-3 fatty acids	proprietary amount

*Total capsules per day can be taken orally, half in the morning and half in the evening with a meal.
[†]Total amounts of antioxidants and herbal products come to 1,870 mg

CONCLUDING REMARKS

As we have learned, several studies on animals and humans suggest that increased levels of oxidative stress, pro-inflammatory cytokines (products of inflammation), and extracellular glutamate in the brain are involved in the progression of damage following penetrating TBI. In order to reduce oxidative stress, chronic inflammation, and glutamate release and its toxicity, it is essential to increase the levels of antioxidant enzymes by activating the Nrf2/ARE pathway. It is also essential to increase the amounts of dietary and endogenous antioxidants in the body at the same time. The above goals cannot be achieved by the utilization of a single antioxidant. Therefore, I have proposed a preparation of micronutrients containing multiple dietary and endogenous antioxidants, and certain polyphenolic compounds (curcumin and resveratrol) and omega-3 fatty acids that would achieve the above goals.

The efficacy of these formulations can be tested in following groups: troops to be employed to the field of combat in order to reduce the initial impact of damage—and in combination with standard therapy, in individuals who have sustained and/or survived penetrating TBI.

Next we will examine PTSD, and determine how a similar formula may be helpful in this instance too.

9 Post-Traumatic Stress Disorder (PTSD)

Causes, Symptoms, Prevalence, and Costs

Humans have been exposed to severe traumatic events for centuries; consequently, individuals have always suffered from the mental disorder we now called post-traumatic stress disorder (PTSD). It wasn't until 1980 that this condition was named as such, when the American Psychiatric Association (APA) included PTSD in its definitive Diagnostic and Statistical Manual of Mental Disorders (DSM-III). The designation of PTSD was remarkable in that it recognized and acknowledged that an external event or events was capable of causing an individual to feel and behave in a traumatized fashion. Prior to this time, the afflicted individual was deemed to be the sole author of the weakened condition they experienced as a result of having been traumatized, whether that traumatization occurred in the field of combat, on the playing field, or in the course of everyday life.

This chapter briefly describes the causes, symptoms, prevalence, and costs of PTSD. It also examines the biochemical defects that help to initiate its development and participate in its progression. In addition, we will cover the studies that have been done to date, which support the hypothesis that increased oxidative stress, chronic inflammation, and glutamate release play an important role in the progression of PTSD.

CAUSES OF PTSD

Post-traumatic stress disorder (PTSD) is a complex condition often caused by an exposure to a blast in a military conflict; sudden or repeatedly extreme traumatic events such as those that occur during war, terrorism, natural- or human-caused disaster; as well as violent personal assault such as rape, mugging, domestic violence, and accidents. There is a strong direct relationship between mild traumatic brain injury (TBI) and PTSD (Hoge et al. 2008; Schneiderman, Braver, and Kang 2008). Several studies have investigated the role of oxidative stress, chronic inflammation, and glutamate release in the progression of PTSD.

SYMPTOMS OF PTSD

Symptoms of PTSD typically appear within three months of the traumatic experience, and often result in a diminished quality of life and considerable emotional suffering for the afflicted individual. Disabling PTSD symptoms include re-experiencing of the trauma memory (flashbacks, nightmares, triggered emotional responses), passive and active avoidance (emotional numbing, avoidance of discussions about the traumatic event), and hyperarousal (sleep problems, concentration problems, irritability, increased startle response, and hypervigilance).

In addition, PTSD is usually accompanied by other psychiatric and medical comorbidities, including depression, substance abuse, cognition dysfunction, and other issues of physical and mental health. In some cases, these symptoms can lead to suicide. It has also been reported that PTSD is associated with general learning impairment as well as memory impairment (Burriss et al. 2008).

These problems generally lead to an impaired ability to function in social and family life and tendencies include job instability and marital and family problems. Some of the symptoms of PTSD may overlap with those of other conditions or diseases such as chronic fatigue syndrome, fibromyalgia, and multiple chemical sensitivity (Pall and Satterlee 2001).

BRAIN DAMAGE IN PTSD

Brain damage in patients with PTSD is not well understood because sufficient amounts of autopsied brain tissue are not available for studying changes in the afflicted brain. Most of the data on brain damage have been obtained by examining brain tissue by MRI (magnetic resonance imaging), a non-invasive technique for studying changes in the brain. The reduction in the volume of certain areas of the brain—particularly the hippocampus, which is responsible for memory—has been consistently observed by this technique.

The fact that a reduced volume of the hippocampus region of the brain was observed by MRI in the brains of patients with PTSD suggests that a significant loss of cholinergic neurons had occurred. This loss could account for the loss of memory (cognitive dysfunction) commonly observed in patients with PTSD (Bremner et al. 1993; Tischler et al. 2006).

Furthermore, an increased rate of brain tissue loss, particularly in the brain stem and frontal and temporal lobes, was associated with an increased severity of PTSD symptoms (Cardenas et al. 2011). In addition, it was observed that the greater the loss of brain tissue, the greater were the declines in verbal memory and delayed facial recognition.

Another MRI study showed that the gray matter abnormalities in the cortex decreased in patients with PTSD compared to that of healthy individuals (Tavanti et al. 2012).

An MRI study on the brains of twins with and without PTSD

revealed that a significant reduction in gray matter volume occurred in certain areas of the brain regions in twins with PTSD compared to twins without PTSD (Kasai et al. 2008).

The cerebellum of the brain is involved in fear perception, anxiety, anticipation of an event, memory recollection, and regulation of emotion. Examination of the brain by MRI showed that reduction in volume of the cerebellum was associated with mood changes, anxiety, and PTSD symptomatology. Reduction in the volume of the vermis was associated with early traumatic life experiences, and may be considered a risk factor for the future development of PTSD (Baldacara et al. 2011).

A review of 9 studies with 319 subjects revealed that reduction in gray matter occurred in certain areas of the brain in PTSD patients compared to individuals exposed to trauma but without symptoms of PTSD (Kuhn and Gallinat 2013).

Serotonin transporter (5-HTT) protein located in the amygdala regulates stress response. Therefore, deficient 5-HTT function and abnormal amygdala activity may contribute to the development of PTSD. This was shown by the fact that PTSD patients exhibited reduced amygdala expression of 5-HTT, as measured by PET (positron emission tomography), using a radioactive tracer of 5-HTT (^{11}C-AFM). It was observed that reduced amygdala 5-HTT binding was associated with higher anxiety and symptoms of depression in PTSD patients (Murrough et al. 2011).

PREVALENCE OF PTSD

Prevalence refers to the total number of people with PTSD in a population at a given time period; incidence refers to the number of people with a new diagnosis of PTSD annually. The U.S. National Comorbidity Survey Replication (NCS-R) estimated that the lifetime prevalence of PTSD among adult Americans was 6.8 percent (Gradus

2011). The lifetime prevalence of PTSD among men was 3.6 percent, and among women 9.7 percent. The one-year prevalence of PTSD among men was estimated to be 1.8 percent in men and 5.2 percent in women. These data suggest that women are more sensitive and more apt to develop PTSD than men after exposure to the precipitating traumatic events.

Children and adolescents who are exposed to at least one traumatic experience such as abuse or natural disaster have a higher prevalence of PTSD than adults in the general population. This is due to the fact that the brains of children are more sensitive to damage by traumatic stress than are the brains of adults. The 6-month prevalence of PTSD among adolescents between the ages of 13–17 was estimated to be 3.7 percent for boys and 6.3 percent for girls (Gradus 2011).

PTSD affects about 7.7 million Americans over the ages of 18 or about 3.5 percent of people in this age group in a given year (Kessler et al. 2005).

In a recent large-scale study of military personnel in current theaters of combat, it was demonstrated that U.S. Army and Marine Corps personnel returning from duty in Iraq exhibited PTSD rates of 18 percent and 20 percent respectively (Hoge et al. 2004).

Before deployment, only 5 percent of soldiers showed PTSD symptoms, but after a full year of deployment about 17 percent of soldiers exhibited PTSD symptoms. The rate of increase in PTSD was proportional to their length of stay in Iraq (Castro 2005) (table 9.1).

Among total Gulf War veterans, the prevalence of PTSD was estimated to be 10.1 percent (Gradus 2011).

The number of soldiers with PTSD may further increase due to repeated combat deployments (Friedman 2005). In 2007, the National Center for Post-traumatic Stress Disorder estimated that the incidence of PTSD among American Vietnam veterans was about 30.9 percent for men and 26.9 percent for women. An additional 22.5 percent of men and 21.2 percent of women have had partial PTSD. This constitutes about 1.7 million Vietnam veterans who have experienced clinically significant combat-related stress disorder.

The table below articulates the prevelance of PTSD among military personnel.

TABLE 9.1. PREVALENCE OF PARTIAL AND FULLY ESTABLISHED PTSD IN U.S. MILITARY PERSONNEL AFTER DEPLOYMENT

Source	Prevalence (percent)
Veterans from Iraq, 2006	18–20
Veterans from Vietnam, 2007	30.9 in men
	26.9 in women
	22.5 partial PTSD in men
	21.2 partial PTSD in women

COSTS OF PTSD

The estimated societal costs of PTSD among troops returning home over a period of two years varied from about $6,000 to more than $25,000 per case. The total costs over the two-year period—including costs of direct medical treatment and care, and costs associated with lost productivity and suicide—ranged from $4 billion to $6.2 billion (Rand Corporation analysis, 2008). In 2010, the Veterans Health Administration (VHA) spent $2 billion (direct medical cost) to treat veterans with PTSD.

BIOCHEMICAL DEFECTS RESPONSIBLE FOR THE PROGRESSION OF PTSD

The biochemical defects responsible for the progression of PTSD include increased oxidative stress and chronic inflammation, and release of glutamate (table 9.2). Another important factor appears to be the inhibition of gamma-aminobutyric acid (GABA) in PTSD that increases activity of glutamate. Although they are not fully understood, these defects can, nevertheless, provide a basis for developing an effective strategy for reducing the debilitating effects of PTSD, and when combined with standard therapy, may improve the management of this condition.

TABLE 9.2. BIOCHEMICAL DEFECTS RESPONSIBLE FOR THE INITIATION AND PROGRESSION OF PTSD

Biochemical Events	Status
Markers of oxidative stress	Increases
Markers of chronic inflammation	Increases
Glutamate release	Increases
Certain gene expression profiles	Altered
Extinction of conditioned fear	Impaired

Evidence of Increased Oxidative Stress in PTSD

In Human Studies

Some human studies indicate that the presence of excessive amounts of free radicals may be involved in the development and progression of several human chronic neurological disorders, including PTSD (Bremner 2006).

Exposure to traumatic stress increases the activity of nitric oxide synthase (NOS) that can generate excessive amounts of nitric oxide (Harvey et al. 2005; Harvey et al. 2004). Oxidation of nitric oxide produces peroxynitrite, which is very toxic to the nerve cells (Pall and Satterlee 2001).

Peroxynitrite can then damage vital molecules such as DNA, RNA, lipids, and other structures in the brain, which may increase the risk of developing PTSD. Indeed, elevated levels of peroxynitrite and its precursor nitric oxide have been observed in patients with PTSD (Tezcan et al. 2003).

The levels of platelet monoamine oxidase, which generate excessive amounts of free radicals while degrading catecholamines (such as dopamine, epinephrine, and norepinephrine), were elevated in patients with PTSD (Richardson 1993).

This is further confirmed by the fact that loss of catecholamines has been observed in patients with PTSD (Pivac et al. 2007). Peroxynitrite and other free radicals increase the level of oxidative damage in the brain of patients with PTSD, causing memory and other brain dysfunctions.

These few studies that have been done in humans support a hypothesis that increased levels of oxidative stress may contribute to the ongoing progression of PTSD and associated cognitive dysfunctions. This has also been confirmed in animal models of PTSD, which are described next.

In Animal Studies

Exposure to stress can induce PTSD-like symptoms in animals. A review has described the impacts of stress, which include sleep deprivation and social isolation (Schiavone et al. 2013).

Rats exposed to a single prolonged stress exhibited symptoms of PTSD. These rats showed apoptosis (cell death) in the hippocampus region of the brain and impaired memory. Rats exposed to foot shock and maternal separation (forms of stress) exhibited impaired spatial memory and increased number of DNA breaks in the hippocampus (Diehl et al. 2012).

It is interesting to point out that increased oxidative stress has been also observed in other neurodegenerative diseases, such as Alzheimer's disease (Prasad, Cole, and Prasad 2002). The attenuation of oxidative stress appears to be one of the rational choices of reducing the progression of PTSD.

Evidence of Increased Chronic Inflammation in PTSD in Human Studies

In addition to increased oxidative stress, increased chronic inflammation due to activation of microglia may be associated with the development of PTSD. For example, serum levels of interleukin-6 (IL-6) are elevated in patients with PTSD (Yehuda 2001).

Increased levels of IL-6 and IL-6 receptors were found in patients with PTSD (Maes et al. 1999).

High levels of tumor necrosis factor-alpha (TNF-alpha) and IL-1beta were elevated in patients with PTSD in comparison to healthy individuals (von Kanel et al. 2007).

Psychological stress induces a chronic inflammatory process (Sutherland, Alexander, and Hutchison 2003).

Chronic fear and terror in women, but not in men, is associated with elevated levels of C-reactive protein (CRP), which may contribute to an increased risk of cardiovascular disease in PTSD patients (Melamed et al. 2004).

The levels of CRP and IL-6 receptors were elevated in patients with PTSD (Miller et al. 2001).

In a clinical study of 35 severely traumatized PTSD patients and 25 healthy individuals, it was demonstrated that spontaneous production of pro-inflammatory cytokines IL-1ß, IL-6, and tumor necrosis factor-alpha (TNF-alpha) by peripheral blood mononuclear cells (PBMCs) was significantly higher in patients with PTSD than in healthy individuals. Furthermore, the increased levels of these pro-inflammatory cytokines correlated with the severity of PTSD symptoms (Gola et al. 2013). However, circulating plasma levels of pro- and anti-inflammatory cytokines, such as IL-6, IL-8, IL-10, TNF-alpha, or monocyte chemotactic protein (MCP)-1 were not significantly changed either in PTSD patients or in healthy individuals. These studies suggest that chronic inflammation is present in patients with PTSD.

In a clinical study of 48 patients with an established pain disorder or PTSD, and 48 age-sex-matched healthy individuals, it was found that the increased levels of pro-inflammatory cytokines were detectable in the serum of 87 percent of patients with anxiety (men and women), but only 25 percent of healthy individuals showed such changes (Hoge et al. 2009).

Another clinical study of 50 patients with PTSD and 50 age-sex-matched healthy individuals demonstrated that the levels of pro-inflammatory cytokines (IL-2, IL-4, IL-6, IL-8, IL-10, and TNF-alpha) were elevated in the serum of patients with PTSD compared to healthy individuals (Guo et al. 2012).

These studies all suggest that increased levels of chronic inflammation may also contribute to the progression of PTSD and associated behavioral and cognitive dysfunctions. Increased chronic inflammation is also associated with certain neurodegenerative diseases such as Alzheimer's disease (Prasad, Cole, and Prasad 2002). Thus, attenuation of chronic inflammation may be something to aim for in the management of this condition and the mitigation of its progression.

Evidence of Increased Glutamate Release in PTSD in Human Studies

Stress-induced increased levels of glutamate in the brain appear to play an important role in the brain damage associated with PTSD (Nair and Singh Ajit 2008).

The effect of glutamate is mediated by increasing the release of corticotropin-releasing factor (CRF). Increased levels of CRF have been found in the cerebral spinal fluid of patients with PTSD (Bremner et al. 1997). Stress-induced glutamate release and glucocorticoids contribute to a reduction in the volume of the hippocampus in patients with PTSD.

Glutamate and nitric oxide (NO) released during stress also play a central role in maintaining anxiety disorders (Nair and Singh Ajit 2008; Harvey et al. 2005). Stress activates glutamate-NMDA receptors and decreases brain-derived neurotrophic factors (BDNF). Excessive amounts of glutamate can cause the death of cholinergic neurons, which may account for the cognitive dysfunction associated with PTSD. Therefore, blocking the release of glutamate and reducing its toxicity in the brain would be useful in reducing the risk of the progression of PTSD symptoms. Indeed, anti-glutamatergic agents such as lamotrigine improve some of the symptoms of PTSD (re-experiencing hyperarousal and avoidance).

Evidence of Inhibition of Gamma-Aminobutyric Acid (GABA) in PTSD in Human Studies

The levels of GABA in the cortex were lower in PTSD patients than in matched healthy individuals. Lower levels of GABA were associated with a higher state of anxiety (Rosso et al. 2013).

Plasma levels of GABA were lower in PTSD patients than in healthy individuals (Vaiva et al. 2006). Lower levels of GABA can enhance the action of glutamate on the degeneration of nerve cells associated with PTSD.

CONCLUDING REMARKS

The debilitating neurological disorder known as post-traumatic stress disorder may ensue as a result of directly experiencing or witnessing a traumatic event. Post-traumatic stress disorder often is a by-product of war, or the result of an accident or criminal event. Its frightening symptoms may include substance abuse, problems with learning and memory, nightmares, cognition dysfunction, reliving of the traumatic event, and hyperarousal, among others.

As we have learned, PTSD affects approximately 7.7 million Americans over the ages of 18. Additionally, its incidence among soldiers and veterans is on the uptick. Typically symptoms of PTSD develop soon after the traumatizing event but often the symptoms surface much later, making its diagnosis even that much more difficult.

As with concussive injury and penetrating traumatic brain injury, there is some evidence in humans and animal models of PTSD to show that increased oxidative stress, chronic inflammation, and glutamate release play an important role in its progression. Therefore, and again, reducing these biochemical defects may be an advisable choice for decreasing the risk of the progression of PTSD.

We will examine PTSD more closely in the following chapter.

10 Treating and Managing PTSD with Vitamins and Antioxidants

Post-traumatic stress disorder (PTSD) is a complex mental health condition that is typically associated with soldiers and the theater of battle, although a myriad of experiences in a variety of settings can be responsible for its onset. PTSD occurs when one experiences or witnesses a terrifying event, and its symptomatology may manifest in a variety of ways.

As regards PTSD among soldiers of war, currently no preventive strategies exist for U.S. troops who are scheduled to be deployed to military engagement or for those who have been exposed to PTSD-related risk factors but have not yet developed the symptoms of or been diagnosed with PTSD. Standard treatment for PTSD involves addressing the symptoms, not its causes. As such, standard treatment typically involves the prescription of antidepressant medications and psychological counseling, both of which are considered unsatisfactory (Hamner, Robert, and Frueh 2004). Thus, in the afflicted individual, the condition continues to develop and progress.

This chapter describes studies on antioxidants and certain polyphenolic compounds in PTSD and goes on to put forth the rationale for using a proposed preparation of micronutrients that would simultaneously reduce oxidative stress, chronic inflammation, and glutamate release and its toxicity in order to improve the management of this disorder.

THE EFFECT OF A SINGLE ANTIOXIDANT IN STUDIES OF PTSD

In Animal Studies

A few animal studies on the effects of antioxidants in PTSD as well as on other neurological conditions are described here.

Omega-3 Fatty Acids

The question arose whether or not supplementation with omega-3 fatty acids during the period of brain development can protect the adult brain against trauma. To answer this question, rats were fed diets enriched with or deficient in omega-3 fatty acids during the period of brain development. After attaining adulthood, rats were switched to a Western diet and then subjected to mild traumatic brain injury to induce PTSD. The result showed the following: Animals that were subjected to mild traumatic brain injury exhibited an increase in anxiety and the neuropeptide Y receptor type 1 (NPY1R), which are characteristics of PTSD (Tyagi et al. 2013). These symptoms were aggravated in rats that were fed a diet that was deficient in omega-3 fatty acids during the period of brain development.

The results suggest that a diet deficient in omega-3 fatty acids during the period of brain development may lower the threshold of certain neurological disorders (such as PTSD), in response to a trauma or accident. These preliminary human and animal studies suggest that omega-3 fatty acids may be of some value in reducing the risk of developing PTSD, however, additional studies are needed to substantiate this observation.

Curcumin

Curcumin is the active ingredient of turmeric, a spice that is widely used throughout the Indian subcontinent. Curcumin exhibits anti-oxidant and anti-inflammatory activities. Administration of curcumin increased the hippocampal neurogenesis (development of neurons) in chronically stressed rats, similar to the effects of treatment with the antidepressant imipramine. These new hippocampal cells mature and become neurons. In addition, curcumin treatment prevented stress-induced decline in the serotonin receptor 1 A (5-HT-1A) mRNA and brain-derived neurotrophic factor (BDNF) protein levels in the brain's hippocampal regions (Xu et al. 2007). 5-HT-1A is important for maintaining normal mood, whereas BDNF protects neurons against toxic agents.

Flavonoids

Flavonoids also exhibit antioxidant and anti-inflammatory activities. Xiaobuxin-Tang (XBXT), a traditional Chinese herbal product, has been used for the treatment of depressive disorders for centuries in China. Flavonoids (XBXT-2) isolated from the extract of XBXT increased neurogenesis in the hippocampus of chronically stressed rats. In addition, this treatment with flavonoids prevented a stress-induced decrease in brain-derived neurotrophic factor (BDNF) (Aarsland et al. 2008)

In Human Studies

The role of antioxidants in the prevention and improved management of PTSD in humans has not been adequately evaluated, although it has been reported that daily supplementation with omega-3 fatty acids reduced some of the symptoms of PTSD in critically injured patients during the earthquake in Japan in 2011 (Matsuoka et al. 2011).

THE EFFECT OF INDIVIDUAL ANTIOXIDANTS AND B VITAMINS ON OTHER NEURODEGENERATIVE DISEASES IN ANIMAL STUDIES

In an MPTP-rat model of Parkinson's disease, the administration of a mixture of dietary and endogenous antioxidants before treatment with MPTP blocked MPTP-induced depletion of tyrosine hydroxylase (TH), an essential enzyme for the formation of dihydroxyphenylamine (DOPA), a precursor of dopamine. In patients with Parkinson's disease, reduction in dopamine is found. MPTP treatment induces Parkinson-like syndrome by reducing dopamine levels. In other words, antioxidant treatment enhanced the levels of dopamine, and thus prevented the MPTP-induced reduction in dopamine. Antioxidants also blocked MPTP-induced hypokinesia (decreased body movements), one of the symptoms of Parkinson's disease.

The studies discussed above suggest that antioxidants have neuroprotective value. They provide a scientific rationale for testing the effectiveness of the proposed micronutrient preparation for reducing the risk of developing PTSD, and in combination with standard therapy, for decreasing the progression of the condition as well as for improving its overall management.

PROPOSED PREVENTION STRATEGIES IN PTSD

Primary Prevention of PTSD

As regards PTSD, it's not feasible to develop a primary prevention strategy, because the traumatic events that increase the risk of developing PTSD typically occur suddenly and without warning. However, in some cases, such as U.S. troops on the verge of being deployed to military fields of battle, it's possible to develop a primary prevention strategy that might increase the threshold for developing PTSD following exposure to PTSD-related risk factors, such as blasts and other traumatic events.

Secondary Prevention of PTSD

Secondary prevention of PTSD targets individuals who may be at risk for developing PTSD but who have not been formally diagnosed with it, nor are they taking medication to mitigate its effects. These persons may be at risk for developing PTSD due to having been exposed to traumatic wartime events. As we have learned, free radical production, inflammation, and glutamate release increases following exposure to the precipitating events of PTSD. These agents are apt to enhance the development of PTSD, thus a logical secondary prevention strategy, as with a primary prevention strategy, is to mitigate the cascading effects of these agents by suppressing their production.

The secondary prevention strategy in combination with standard care should begin soon after an individual has been exposed to PTSD-related risk factors.

Recommended Micronutrients in
Secondary Prevention of PTSD
The doses of all recommended micronutrients are listed in table 10.1.

Standard Therapy in
Secondary Prevention of PTSD
The purpose of standard therapy is to slow the progression of the condition and improve its symptoms. Standard therapy includes the administration of drugs and psychological/psychiatric counseling. As mentioned earlier, drug therapy is primarily based on the symptoms rather than the causes of PTSD.

TABLE 10.1. INGREDIENTS OF A RECOMMENDED MICRONUTRIENT PREPARATION FOR PRIMARY AND SECONDARY PREVENTION OF PTSD (DAILY DOSES)*

Vitamin A (retinyl palmitate)	3,000 IU
Natural vitamin E	400 IU (d-alpha-tocopherol succinate 250 IU) (d-alpha-tocopheryl acetate 150 IU)
Vitamin C (calcium ascorbate)	1,000 mg
Vitamin D$_3$ (cholecalciferol)	1,000 IU
Vitamin B$_1$ (thiamine mononitrate)	10 mg
Vitamin B$_2$ (riboflavin)	4 mg
Vitamin B$_3$ (nicotinamide)	100 mg
Vitamin B$_6$ (pyridoxine hydrochloride)	4 mg
Folic acid(as folate)	400 mcg
Vitamin B$_{12}$ (methylcobalamln)	100 mcg
Biotin	150 mcg
Pantothenic acid (d-calcium pantothenate)	15 mg
Zinc glycinate	5 mg
Selenium (seleno-L-methionine)	100 mcg
N-acetylcysteine (NAC)	proprietary amount†
Coenzyme Q10	proprietary amount
R-alpha-lipoic acid	proprietary amount
L-carnitine	proprietary amount
Resveratrol	proprietary amount
Curcumin	proprietary amount
Omega-3 fatty acids	proprietary amount

*Total capsules per day can be taken orally, half in the morning and half in the evening with a meal.
†Total amounts of antioxidants and herbal products come to 1,585 mg

Standard therapy has produced very limited success in the treatment of PTSD: None of the drugs used in its treatment affect the levels of increased oxidative stress and chronic inflammation that play an important role in the progression of this condition. Therefore, additional approaches that could improve the management of PTSD and reduce its progression should be developed.

Some examples of commonly used medications to improve the symptoms of PTSD are described below. More detailed information on these substances can be found on the website of the United States Department of Veterans Affairs (www.va.gov/) (National Center for PTSD, 2013).

Selective serotonin reuptake inhibitors (SSRIs): Serotonin is important in regulating several body functions including mood, anxiety, appetite, and sleep. Examples of SSRIs are sertraline (Zoloft), paroxetine (Paxil), and fluoxetine (Prozac). Selective serotonin reuptake inhibitors also were useful in improving the symptoms of PTSD (Ipser, Seedat, and Stein 2006).

Antidepressants: Examples of antidepressants are mirtazapine (Remeron), venlafaxine (Effexor), and Nefazodone (Serzone).

Mood stabilizers: These medications are also called anticonvulsants or antiepileptic drugs. They block glutamate release or enhance GABA release or both. Mood stabilizer drugs include carbamazepine (Tegretol), divalproex (Depakote), Lamotrigine (Lamictal), and topiramate (Topimax).

Benzodiazepines: These drugs directly act on the GABA system, which produces calming effects on the central nervous system, but they are potentially addictive and not very effective in treating the core symptoms of PTSD. Examples of benzodiazepines are lorazepam (Ativan), clonazepam (klonopin), and alprazolam (Xanax).

D-cycloserine: Extinction of conditioned fear appears to be defective in patients with PTSD. D-cycloserine, a partial agonist of the NMDA receptor, was useful in enhancing extinction of learned fear in rats (Richardson, Ledgerwood, and Cranney 2004).

This was achieved when d-cycloserine was administered shortly before or after the extinction training of rats (Vervliet 2008). Additionally, in a 6-week randomized, double-blind, placebo-controlled trial using 22 chronic PTSD outpatients, it was found that d-serine, an endogenous agonist of the NMDA receptor at the site of glycine, may improve some of the symptoms of PTSD (Heresco-Levy et al. 2009). The anti-glutamatergic agent lamotrigine was also effective in reducing some of the symptoms of PTSD (Nair and Singh Ajit 2008).

Cortisol: Persistent retrieval and maintenance of traumatic memories is a biological process that keeps these memories vivid and thereby maintains the symptoms of PTSD. It has been demonstrated that elevated glucocorticoid levels inhibit the memory retrieval process in animals and humans (de Quervain and Margraf 2008).

In patients with PTSD, low-dose cortisol treatment for one month reduced symptoms of traumatic memories without causing adverse health effects, probably by preventing the recall of traumatic memories (de Quervain and Margraf 2008; Schelling 2002).

Other medications: Some examples are prazosin (Minipress), tricyclic antidepressants (imipramine), and monoamine oxidase inhibitors (Phenelzine).

The efficacy of drugs in the treatment of PTSD, such as antidepressants, anti-adrenergic agents, anticonvulsants, benzodiazepines, and atypical antipsychotics yielding variable degrees of improvement, has been reviewed (Ravindran and Stein 2009).

None of the drugs that are currently used in the treatment of PTSD decreased the oxidative stress and chronic inflammation that play such an important role in its progression. Therefore, we propose a novel micronutrient strategy that, in combination with standard therapy, may further improve the symptoms of PTSD and slow down its rate of progression.

Recommended Micronutrients in Combination with Standard Therapy in Secondary Prevention of PTSD

As we know, the current standard therapies are not considered sufficient in the management of PTSD. The use of the proposed micronutrient preparation in combination with standard therapy may improve the management of PTSD and reduce the progression of PTSD more than that produced by standard therapy alone.

Diet and Lifestyle Recommendations for PTSD

In addition to supplementation with the proposed micronutrient preparation, a balanced diet low in fat and high in fiber and rich in fruits and vegetables is necessary for reducing the risk of developing PTSD, as well as for improving the effectiveness of standard therapy in its management. Lifestyle recommendations include moderate daily exercise, reduced stress, no smoking, and a reduced intake of caffeine and alcoholic beverages.

CONCLUDING REMARKS

In this chapter we have explored the human and animal studies that have been undertaken to understand more about the neurological condition known as post-traumatic stress disorder (PTSD). As we have ascertained, currently, no preventive strategies exist to reduce the risk of its development and the current standard therapy for treating it—drug therapy and psychological counseling—is considered unsatisfactory in large part because this protocol addresses the symptoms of PTSD, not its causes.

As we know, the major biochemical defects that contribute to the progression of PTSD include increased oxidative stress, chronic inflammation, and the release of glutamate. These biochemical defects are not impacted by current standard therapy, thus PTSD and its associated concerns continue to escalate.

Again, as with concussive injury and penetrating TBI, an elevation of all antioxidant enzymes and all dietary and endogenous antioxidants is necessary for optimally reducing these defects of oxidative stress, chronic inflammation, and the release of glutamate.

The micronutrient preparation that I recommend, which contains multiple dietary and endogenous antioxidants and certain polyphenolic compounds (curcumin and resveratrol), and omega-3 fatty acids, may be sufficient to achieve this objective. This is due to the fact that it is capable of activating the Nrf2/ARE regulated pathway, which increases the levels of antioxidant enzymes as well as enhancing the levels of dietary and endogenous antioxidants at the same time.

This proposed micronutrient preparation may be adopted by troops who are about to be deployed to a theater of battle or to individuals who have been exposed to traumatic stressors but who have not developed the symptoms of PTSD. Additionally, these recommendations may be adopted by those individuals who have been diagnosed with PTSD and are on standard care in consulatation with their doctors. It is expected that those who currently suffer from its debilitating effects find that micronutrient strategy may help them better manage this insidious condition.

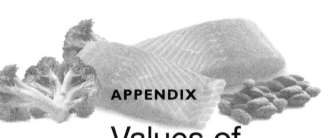

Values of Recommended Dietary Allowances (RDA)/ Dietary Reference Intakes (DRI)

Note to the Reader: All of the information contained in this appendix, including the tables, is from my book *Fighting Cancer with Vitamins and Antioxidants,* coauthored with my son K. C. Prasad, M.S., M.D., published by Healing Arts Press in 2011.

■ ■ ■

Sufficient changes in nutritional guidelines have occurred since World War II due to increased knowledge of nutrition and health. The nutritional guidelines referred to as Recommended Dietary Allowances (RDAs) were first established in 1941. The Food and Nutrition Board of the United States subsequently revise these guidelines every five to ten years.

RDA (DRI)

RDA refers to the value of the daily dietary intake level of a nutrient considered sufficient to meet the requirements of 97 to 98 percent of healthy individuals of different ages and genders. Because of the rapid growth of research on the role of nutrients in human health, the Food and Nutrition Board of the Institute of Medicine (IOM) of the United States in collaboration with Health Canada updated the values of RDAs and renamed them Dietary Reference Intakes (DRIs) in 1998. Since then DRIs values have been used by both the United States and Canada. The DRI values of selected nutrients are listed in tables A.1 to A.21. The DRI values are not currently used in nutrition labeling; the RDA values of nutrients continue to be used for this purpose. The DRI values for carotenoids, alpha-lipoic acid, n-acetylcysteine, coenzyme Q10 and L-carnitine have not been determined.

ADEQUATE INTAKE (AI)

Adequate intake refers to the value of a nutrient for which no RDA has been established, but the value established may be sufficient for everyone in the demographic group.

TOLERABLE UPPER INTAKE LEVEL (UL)

The tolerable upper intake level is the maximum level of daily nutrient intake that is likely to pose no risk of adverse health effects. The UL value represents total intake of a nutrient from food, water, and supplements.

RELATIONSHIP BETWEEN RECOMMENDED DIETARY ALLOWANCES VALUES AND OPTIMAL HEALTH

RDA values of nutrients are expected to be adequate for individuals for normal growth and survival, however, the values of micronutrients needed for prevention or improved management of human diseases are not known at this time. The data on doses obtained from the use of a single micronutrient in the prevention or treatment of neurological conditions should not be extrapolated to the doses of the same micronutrient present in a multiple micronutrient preparation.

RDA/DRI values of micronutrients are sufficient for normal growth and survival, but they are not adequate for prevention or improved treatment of human diseases. In order to evaluate the dosage of micronutrients in any multivitamin preparation for the prevention or improved treatment of neurological conditions, it is essential to have sufficient knowledge of the RDA values of the micronutrients as found in the next section of this book.

CONCLUDING REMARKS

The initial nutritional guidelines, Recommended Dietary Allowances (RDAs), have been replaced by Dietary Reference Intakes (DRIs), and are currently used in the United States and Canada. The DRI values of nutrients are sufficient for the growth and development of 97 to 98 percent of healthy individuals. The DRI values for carotenoids, alpha-lipoic acid, N-acetylcysteine, coenzyme Q10, and L-carnitine have not been determined. The optimal values needed for the prevention or improved management of Alzheimer's disease is not known. Both preventive and therapeutic doses of micronutrients are higher than their RDA values.

TABLE A.1. DIETARY REFERENCE
INTAKES (DRI) OF ANTIOXIDANT VITAMIN A

Age	RDA/AI*	UL
	µg/d (IU/d)	µg/d (IU/d)
Infants		
0–6 mo	400 (1,200 IU)*	600 (1,800 IU)
7–12 mo	500 (1,500 IU)*	600 (1,800 IU)
Children		
1–3 y	300 (900 IU)	600 (1,800 IU)
4–8 y	400 (1,200 IU)	900 (2,700 IU)
Males		
9–13 y	600 (1,800 IU)	1,700 (5,100 IU)
14–18 y	900 (2,700 IU)	2,800 (8,400 IU)
19 y and up	900 (2,700 IU)	3,000 (9,000 IU)
Females		
9–13 y	600 (1,800 IU)	1,700 (5,100 IU)
14–18 y	700 (2,100 IU)	2,800 (8,400 IU)
19 y and up	700 (2,100 IU)	3,000 (9,000 IU)
Pregnancy		
under 18 y	750 (2,250 IU)	2,800 (8,400 IU)
19–50 y	770 (2,310 IU)	3,000 (9,000 IU)
Lactation		
under 18 y	1,200 (3,600 IU)	2,800 (8,400 IU)
19–50 y	1,300 (3,900 IU)	3,000 (9,000 IU)

1 µg of retinol equals 1 µg of RAE (retinol activity equivalent); 1 IU of retinol equals 0.3 µg of retinol; and 2 µg of beta-carotene equals 1 µg of retinol.

RDA = Recommended Dietary Allowances
*AI = Adequate Intake
UL = Tolerable Upper Intake Value
µg = microgram; d = day

The values are adapted and summarized from the table of the Dietary Reference Intakes (DRI) published by www.nap.edu. (Search on "Food and Nutrition" and you will find information about DRI.)

TABLE A.2. DIETARY REFERENCE
INTAKES (DRI) OF ANTIOXIDANT VITAMIN C

Age	RDA/AI*	UL
	mg/d	mg/d
Infants		
0–6 mo	40*	ND
7–12 mo	50*	ND
Children		
1–3 y	15	400
4–8 y	25	650
Males		
9–13 y	45	1,200
14–18 y	75	1,800
19 y and up	90	2,000
Females		
9–13 y	45	1,200
14–18 y	65	1,800
19 y and up	75	2,000

RDA = Recommended Dietary Allowances
*AI = Adequate Intake
UL = Tolerable Upper Intake Value
μg = microgram; d = day

The values are adapted and summarized from the table of the Dietary Reference Intakes (DRI) published by www.nap.edu.

TABLE A.3. DIETARY REFERENCE
INTAKES (DRI) OF ANTIOXIDANT VITAMIN E

Age	RDA/AI*	UL
	mg/d (IU/d)	mg/d (IU/d)
Infants		
0–6 mo	4 (6 IU)*	ND
7–12 mo	5 (7.5 IU)*	ND
Children		
1–3 y	6 (9 IU)	200 (30 IU)
4–8 y	7 (10.6 IU)	300 (45 IU)
Males		
9–13 y	11 (16.7 IU)	600 (90 IU)
14–18 y	15 (22.8 IU)	800 (120 IU)
19 y and up	15 (22.8 IU)	1,000 (150 IU)
Females		
9–13 y	11 (16.7 IU)	600 (90 IU)
14–18 y	15 (22.8 IU)	800 (120 IU)
19 y and up	15 (22.8 IU)	1,000 (150 IU)
Pregnancy		
under 18 y	15 (22.8 IU)	800 (120 IU)
19–50 y	15 (22.8 IU)	1,000 (150 IU)
Lactation		
under 18 y	19 (28.9 IU)	800 (120 IU)
19–50 y	19 (28.9 IU)	1,000 (150 IU)

RDA = Recommended Dietary Allowances
*AI = Adequate Intake
UL = Tolerable Upper Intake Value
ND = not determined
mg = milligram; d = day
1 IU of vitamin E equals 0.66 mg of d- and 0.45 mg of
dl-alpha-tocopherol.

The values are adapted and summarized from the tables of the Dietary Reference Intakes (DRI)
published by www.nap.edu.

TABLE A.4. DIETARY REFERENCE
INTAKES (DRI) OF VITAMIN D

Age	RDA/AI*	UL
	µg/d (IU/d)	µg/d (IU/d)
Infants		
0–12 mo	5 (200 IU)*	25 (1,000 IU)
Children		
1–8 y	5 (200 IU)*	50 (2,000 IU)
Males		
9–50 y	5 (200 IU)*	50 (2,000 IU)
50–70 y	10 (400 IU)*	50 (2,000 IU)
over 70 y	15 (600 IU)*	50 (2,000 IU)
Females		
9–50 y	5 (200 IU)*	50 (2,000 IU)
50–70 y	10 (400 IU)*	50 (2,000 IU)
under 70 y	15 (600 IU)*	50 (2,000 IU)
Pregnancy		
18–50 y	5 (200 IU)*	50 (2,000 IU)
Lactation		
18–50 y	5 (200 IU)*	50 (2,000 IU)

RDA = Recommended Dietary Allowances
*AI = Adequate Intake
UL = Tolerable Upper Intake Value
µg = microgram; d = day
1 µg of cholecalciferol equals 40 IU (international unit)
of Vitamin D.

The values are adapted and summarized from the tables of the Dietary Reference Intakes (DRI)
published by www.nap.edu.

TABLE A.5. DIETARY REFERENCE
INTAKES (DRI) OF VITAMIN B₁ (THIAMINE)

Age	RDA/AI*	UL
	mg/d	mg/d
Infants		
0–6 mo	0.2*	ND
7–12 mo	0.3*	ND
Children		
1–3 y	0.5	ND
4–8 y	0.6	ND
Males		
9–13 y	0.9	ND
14 y and up	1.2	ND
Females		
9–13 y	0.9	ND
14–18 y	1.0	ND
19 y and up	1.1	ND
Pregnancy		
18–50 y	1.4	ND
Lactation		
18–50 y	1.4	ND

RDA = Recommended Dietary Allowances
*AI = Adequate Intake
UL = Tolerable Upper Intake Value
ND = not determined
mg = milligram; d = day

The values are adapted and summarized from the tables of the Dietary Reference Intakes (DRI) published by www.nap.edu.

TABLE A.6. DIETARY REFERENCE
INTAKES (DRI) OF VITAMIN B₂ (RIBOFLAVIN)

Age	RDA/AI*	UL
	mg/d	mg/d
Infants		
0–6 mo	0.3*	ND
7–12 mo	0.4*	ND
Children		
1–3 y	0.5	ND
4–8 y	0.6	ND
Males		
9–13 y	0.9	ND
14 y and up	13	ND
Females		
9–13 y	0.9	ND
14–18 y	1.0	ND
19 y and up	1.1	ND
Pregnancy		
18–50 y	1.4	ND
Lactation		
18–50 y	1.6	ND

RDA = Recommended Dietary Allowances
*AI = Adequate Intake
UL = Tolerable Upper Intake Value
ND = not determined
mg = milligram; d = day

The values are adapted and summarized from the table of the Dietary Reference Intakes (DRI) published by www.nap.edu.

TABLE A.7. DIETARY REFERENCE
INTAKES (DRI) OF VITAMIN B₆

Age	RDA/AI*	UL
	mg/d	mg/d
Infants		
0–6 mo	0.1*	ND
7–12 mo	0.3*	ND
Children		
1–3 y	0.5	30
4–8 y	0.6	40
Males		
9–13 y	1.0	60
14–50 y	1.3	80
50–70 y and up	1.7	100
Females		
9–13 y	1.0	60
14–18 y	1.2	80
19–30 y	1.3	100
50 y and up	1.5	100
Pregnancy		
under 18 y	1.9	80
19–50 y	1.9	100
Lactation		
under 18 y	2.0	80
19–50 y	2.0	100

RDA = Recommended Dietary Allowances
*AI = Adequate Intake
UL = Tolerable Upper Intake Value
ND = not determined
mg = milligram; d = day

The values are adapted and summarized from the table of the Dietary Reference Intakes (DRI) published by www.nap.edu.

TABLE A.8. DIETARY REFERENCE
INTAKES (DRI) OF VITAMIN B₁₂ (COBALAMIN)

Age	RDA/AI*	UL
	µg/d	µg/d
Infants		
0–6 mo	0.4*	ND
7–12 mo	0.5*	ND
Children		
1–3 y	0.9	ND
4–8 y	1.2	ND
Males		
9–13 y	1.08	ND
14 y and up	2.4	ND
Females		
9–13 y	1.8	ND
14 y and up	2.4	ND
Pregnancy		
18–50 y	2.6	ND
Lactation		
18–50 y	2.8	ND

RDA = Recommended Dietary Allowances
*AI = Adequate Intake
UL = Tolerable Upper Intake Value
ND = not determined
µg = microgram; d = day

The values are adapted and summarized from the table of the Dietary Reference Intakes (DRI) published by www.nap.edu.

TABLE A.9. DIETARY REFERENCE
INTAKES (DRI) OF VITAMIN PANTOTHENIC ACID

Age	RDA/AI*	UL
	mg/d	mg/d
Infants		
0–6 mo	1.7*	ND
7–12 mo	1.8*	ND
Children		
1–3 y	2*	ND
4–8 y	2*	ND
Males		
9–13 y	4*	ND
14 y and up	5*	ND
Females		
9–13 y	4*	ND
14 y and up	5*	ND
Pregnancy		
18–50 y	6*	ND
Lactation		
18–50 y	7*	ND

RDA = Recommended Dietary Allowances
*AI = Adequate Intake
UL = Tolerable Upper Intake Value
ND = not determined
mg = milligram; d = day

The values are adapted and summarized from the table of the Dietary Reference Intakes (DRI) published by www.nap.edu.

TABLE A.10. DIETARY REFERENCE
INTAKES (DRI) OF VITAMIN NIACIN

Age	RDA/AI*	UL
	mg/d	mg/d
Infants		
0–6 mo	2*	ND
7–12 mo	0.4*	ND
Children		
1–3 y	6.0	10
4–8 y	8.0	15
Males		
9–13 y	12	20
14–50 y	16	30
50 y and up	16	35
Females		
9–13 y	12	20
14–18 y	14	30
19 y and up	14	35
Pregnancy		
under 18 y	18	30
19–50 y	18	35
Lactation		
under 18 y	17	30
19–50 y	17	35

RDA = Recommended Dietary Allowances
*AI = Adequate Intake
UL = Tolerable Upper Intake Value
ND = not determined
mg = milligram; d = day

The values are adapted and summarized from the table of the Dietary Reference Intakes (DRI) published by www.nap.edu

TABLE A.11. DIETARY REFERENCE
INTAKES (DRI) OF VITAMIN FOLATE

Age	RDA/AI*	UL
	µg/d	µg/d
Infants		
0–6 mo	65*	ND
7–12 mo	80*	ND
Children		
1–3 y	150	300
4–8 y	200	400
Males		
9–13 y	300	600
14–18 y	400	800
19 y and up	400	1,000
Females		
9–13 y	300	600
14–18 y	400	800
19 y and up	400	1,000
Pregnancy		
under 18 y	600	800
19–50 y	600	1,000
Lactation		
under 18 y	500	800
19–50 y	500	1,000

RDA = Recommended Dietary Allowances
*AI = Adequate Intake
UL = Tolerable Upper Intake Value
ND = not determined
µg = microgram; d = day

The values are adapted and summarized from the table of the Dietary Reference Intakes (DRI) published by www.nap.edu.

TABLE A.12. DIETARY REFERENCE
INTAKES (DRI) OF MICRONUTRIENT BIOTIN

Age	RDA/AI*	UL
	µg/d	µg/d
Infants		
0–6 mo	0.5*	ND
7–12 mo	0.6*	ND
Children		
1–3 y	8*	ND
4–8 y	12*	ND
Males		
9–13 y	20	ND
14–18 y	25	ND
19 y and up	30	ND
Females		
9–13 y	20	ND
14–18 y	25	ND
19 y and up	30	ND
Pregnancy		
under 18 y	30*	ND
19–50 y	30*	ND
Lactation		
under 18 y	35*	ND
19–50 y	35*	ND

RDA = Recommended Dietary Allowances
*AI = Adequate Intake
UL = Tolerable Upper Intake Value
ND = not determined
µg = microgram; d = day

The values are adapted and summarized from the table of the Dietary Reference Intakes (DRI) published by www.nap.edu.

TABLE A.13. DIETARY REFERENCE
INTAKES (DRI) OF MINERAL CALCIUM

Age	RDA/AI*	UL
	mg/d	mg/d
Infants		
0–6 mo	210*	ND
7–12 mo	270*	ND
Children		
1–3 y	500*	2,500
4–8 y	800*	2,500
Males		
9–18 y	1,300*	2,500
19–50 y	1,000*	2,500
51 y and up	1,200*	2,500
Females		
9–8 y	1,300*	2,500
19–50 y	1,000*	2,500
51 y and up	1,200*	2,500
Pregnancy		
under 18 y	1,300*	2,500
19–50 y	1,000*	2,500
Lactation		
under 18 y	1,300*	2,500
19–50 y	1,000*	2,500

RDA = Recommended Dietary Allowances
*AI = Adequate Intake
UL = Tolerable Upper Intake Value
ND = not determined
mg = milligram; d = day

The values are adapted and summarized from the table of the Dietary Reference Intakes (DRI) published by www.nap.edu.

TABLE A.14. DIETARY REFERENCE
INTAKES (DRI) OF MINERAL MAGNESIUM

Age	RDA/AI*	UL
	mg/d	mg/d
Infants		
0–6 mo	30*	ND
7–12 mo	75*	ND
Children		
1–3 y	80	65
4–8 y	130	110
Males		
9–13 y	240	350
14–18 y	410	350
19–30 y	400	350
31 y and up	420	350
Females		
9–13 y	240	350
14–18 y	360	350
31 y and up	320	350
Pregnancy		
under 18 y	400	350
19–30 y	350	350
31–50 y	360	350
Lactation		
under 18 y	360	350
31–50 y	320	350

RDA = Recommended Dietary Allowances
*AI = Adequate Intake
UL = Tolerable Upper Intake Value
ND = not determined
mg = milligram; d = day

The values are adapted and summarized from the table of the Dietary Reference Intakes (DRI) published by www.nap.edu.

TABLE A.15. DIETARY REFERENCE
INTAKES (DRI) OF MINERAL MANGANESE

Age	RDA/AI*	UL
	mg/d	mg/d
Infants		
0–6 mo	0.003*	ND
7–12 mo	0.6*	ND
Children		
1–3 y	1.2*	2
4–8 y	1.5*	3
Males		
9–13 y	1.9*	6
14–18 y	2.2*	9
19 y and up	2.3*	11
Females		
9–13 y	1.6*	6
14–18 y	1.6*	9
19 y and up	1.8*	11
Pregnancy		
under 18 y	2.0*	9
19–50 y	2.0*	11
Lactation		
under 18 y	2.6*	9
19–50 y	2.6*	11

RDA = Recommended Dietary Allowances
*AI = Adequate Intake
UL = Tolerable Upper Intake Value
ND = not determined
mg = milligram; d = day

The values are adapted and summarized from the table of the Dietary Reference Intakes (DRI) published by www.nap.edu.

TABLE A.16. DIETARY REFERENCE
INTAKES (DRI) OF MINERAL CHROMIUM

Age	RDA/AI*	UL
	µg/d	µg/d
Infants		
0–6 mo	0.2*	ND
7–12 mo	5.5*	ND
Children		
1–3 y	11*	ND
4–8 y	15*	ND
Males		
9–13 y	25*	ND
14–50 y	35*	ND
51 y and up	30*	ND
Females		
9–13 y	21*	ND
14–18 y	24*	ND
19–50 y	25*	ND
Pregnancy		
under 18 y	29*	ND
19–50 y	30*	ND
Lactation		
under 18 y	44*	ND
19–50 y	45*	ND

RDA = Recommended Dietary Allowances
*AI = Adequate Intake
UL = Tolerable Upper Intake Value
ND = not determined
µg = microgram; d = day

The values are adapted and summarized from the table of the Dietary Reference Intakes (DRI)
published by www.nap.edu.

TABLE A.17. DIETARY REFERENCE
INTAKES (DRI) OF MINERAL COPPER

Age	RDA/AI*	UL
	µg/d	µg/d
Infants		
0–6 mo	200*	ND
7–12 mo	220*	ND
Children		
1–3 y	340	1,000
4–8 y	440	3,000
Males		
9–13 y	700	5,000
14–18 y	890	8,000
19 y and up	900	10,000
Females		
9–13 y	700	5,000
14–18 y	890	8,000
19 y and up	900	10,000
Pregnancy		
under 18 y	1,000	8,000
19–50 y	1,000	10,000
Lactation		
under 18 y	1,300	8,000
19–50 y	1,300	10,000

RDA = Recommended Dietary Allowances
*AI = Adequate Intake
UL = Tolerable Upper Intake Value
ND = not determined
µg = microgram; d = day

The values are adapted and summarized from the table of the Dietary Reference Intakes (DRI) published by www.nap.edu.

TABLE A.18. DIETARY REFERENCE INTAKES (DRI) OF MINERAL IRON

Age	RDA/AI*	UL
	mg/d	mg/d
Infants		
0–6 mo	0.27*	40
7–12 mo	11	40
Children		
1–3 y	7	40
4–8 y	10	40
Males		
9–13 y	8	40
14–18 y	11	45
19 y and up	8	45
Females		
9–13 y	8	40
14–18 y	15	45
19–50 y	18	45
50 y and up	8	45
Pregnancy		
18–50 y	27	45
Lactation		
under 18 y	10	45
19–50 y	9	45

RDA = Recommended Dietary Allowances
*AI = Adequate Intake
UL = Tolerable Upper Intake Value
ND = not determined
mg = milligram; d = day

The values are adapted and summarized from the table of the Dietary Reference Intakes (DRI) published by www.nap.edu.

TABLE A.19. DIETARY REFERENCE
INTAKES (DRI) OF MINERAL SELENIUM

Age	RDA/AI*	UL
	µg/d	µg/d
Infants		
0–6 mo	15*	45
7–12 mo	20*	60
Children		
1–3 y	20	90
4–8 y	30	150
Males		
9–13 y	40	280
14 y and up	55	400
Females		
9–13 y	40	280
14 y and up	55	400
Pregnancy		
18–50 y	60	400
Lactation		
18–50 y	70	400

RDA = Recommended Dietary Allowances
*AI = Adequate Intake
UL = Tolerable Upper Intake Value
ND = not determined
µg = microgram; d = day

The values are adapted and summarized from the table of the Dietary Reference Intakes (DRI) published by www.nap.edu.

TABLE A.20. DIETARY REFERENCE INTAKES (DRI) OF MINERAL PHOSPHORUS

Age	RDA/AI*	UL
	mg/d	mg/d
Infants		
0–6 mo	100*	ND
7–12 mo	275*	ND
Children		
1–3 y	460	3,000
4–8 y	500	3,000
Males		
9–18 y	1,250	4,000
19–70 y	700	4,000
70 y and up	700	3,000
Females		
9–18 y	1,250	4,000
19–70 y	700	4,000
70 y and up	700	3,000
Pregnancy		
under 18 y	1,250	3,500
19–50 y	700	3,500
Lactation		
under 18 y	1,250	4,000
19–50 y	700	4,000

RDA = Recommended Dietary Allowances
*AI = Adequate Intake
UL = Tolerable Upper Intake Value
ND = not determined
mg = milligram; d = day

The values are adapted and summarized from the table of the Dietary Reference Intakes (DRI) published by www.nap.edu.

TABLE A.21. DIETARY REFERENCE
INTAKES (DRI) OF MINERAL ZINC

Age	RDA/AI*	UL
	mg/d	mg/d
Infants		
0–6	2*	4
7–12 mo	3	5
Children		
1–3 y	3	7
4–8 y	5	12
Males		
9–13 y	8	23
14–18 y	11	34
19 y and up	11	40
Females		
9–13 y	8	23
14–18 y	9	34
19 y and up	8	40
Pregnancy		
under 18 y	12	34
19–50 y	11	40
Lactation		
under 18 y	13	34
19–50 y	12	40

RDA = Recommended Dietary Allowances
*AI = Adequate Intake
UL = Tolerable Upper Intake Value
ND = not determined
mg = milligram; d = day

The values are adapted and summarized from the table of the Dietary Reference Intakes (DRI) published by www.nap.edu.

TABLE A.22. CALORIE CONTENT
OF SELECTED FOODS

Food	Portion size	Calories
Apple	1	80
Banana	1	100
Beans, green cooked	½ cup	18
Bread, whole wheat	1 slice	56
Butter	1 tablespoon	100
Carrot	1 medium	34
Cheese	1 ounce	107–114
Corn on the cob	5½ inches	160
Egg	1 large	80
Ice cream	½ cup	135
Kidney beans, cooked	½ cup	110
Meat	3 ounces	200–250
Milk, skim	1 cup	85
Milk, whole	1 cup	150
Orange	1	65
Peach	1	38
Peanuts	1 ounce	172
Pear	1	100
Peas	½ cup	86
Potato chips	10 chips	115
Rice, cooked	½ cup	110
Shrimp	3 ounces	78
Tuna	3 ounces	78
Yogurt, low fat	1 cup	140

From K. N. Prasad and K. C. Prasad, *Fight Cancer with Vitamins and Supplements: A Guide to Prevention and Treatment*, Rochester, Vt.: Healing Arts Press, 2001.

TABLE A.23. FAT CONTENT
OF SELECTED FOODS

Food	Portion size	Grams/Portion
Avocado	⅛	4
Bacon, crisp	2 slices	6
Beef, roast	3 ounces	26
Biscuit	1	4
Bread, whole wheat	1 slice	1
Cheese, cheddar	1 ounce	9
Chicken, baked, with skin	3 ounces	11
Chicken, baked, without skin	3 ounces	6
Cornbread	1 piece	7
Egg, boiled	1	6
Ice cream	½ cup	7
Margarine	1 teaspoon	4
Mayonnaise	1 tablespoon	11
Milk, skim	1 cup	1
Milk, whole	1 cup	8
Oatmeal, cooked	½ cup	1
Peanut butter	1 tablespoon	7
Pork chop	3 ounces	19
Shrimp	3 ounces	0.9
Sour cream	1 tablespoon	3
Tuna	3 ounces	0.9
Vegetable oil	1 teaspoon	5
Yogurt, low fat	1 cup	4

From K. N. Prasad and K. C. Prasad, *Fight Cancer with Vitamins and Supplements: A Guide to Prevention and Treatment*, Rochester, Vt.: Healing Arts Press, 2001.

TABLE A.24. FIBER CONTENT
OF SELECTED FOODS

Food	Portion size	Grams/Portion
Apple, with skin	1	3
Bread, white	1 slice	0.8
Bread, whole wheat	1 slice	1.3
Broccoli	½ cup	3.2
Carrot, raw	1 medium	2.4
Cereal, all-bran	1 cup	25.6
Cereal, raisin bran	1 cup	6
Corn	½ cup	4.6
Muffin, bran	1	4.2
Pear, with skin	1	3.8
Raspberries	½ cup	4.6

From K. N. Prasad and K. C. Prasad, *Fight Cancer with Vitamins and Supplements: A Guide to Prevention and Treatment*, Rochester, Vt.: Healing Arts Press, 2001.

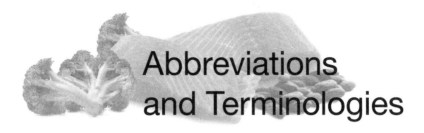

Abbreviations and Terminologies

Aß1-42: Beta-amyloid fragments generated from APPP

APOE: Apolipoprotein E

APP: Amyloid precursor protein

ARE: Antioxidant response element

BDNF: Brain-derived neurotrophic factor

COX: Cyclooxygenase

CRP: C-reactive protein

CSF: Cerebrospinal fluid

DA: Dopamine

GABA: Gamma-aminobutyric acid

GDNF: Glia cell-derived neurotrophic factor

GLT-1: Glutamate transporter-1

GPX: Glutathione peroxidase

H2O2: Hydrogen peroxide

4-HNE: 4-Hydroxynonenal

8-OHdG: 8-Hydroxy-2-deoxyguanosine

HO-1: Heme oxygenase

IED: Improvised explosive device

IL-6: Interleukin-6

MAO: Monoamine oxidase

MCI: Mild cognitive impairment

MDA: Malondialdehyde

MPTP: 1-Methyl-4-phenyl 1,2,3,6-tetrahydropyridine

MRI: Magnetic resonance imaging

mTBI: mild traumatic brain injury or concussive injury

NAC: N-acetylcysteine

NAD: Nicotinamide adenine dinucleotide

NADH: Reduced form of NAD

NFkappaB: Nuclear factor kappa-beta

NGF: Nerve growth factor

NMDA: N-methy-D-aspartate

NO: Nitric oxide

Nrf2: Nuclear factor-erythroid 2-related factor 2

3-NT: 3-Nitrotyrosine

PAMARA: Protection as much as reasonably achievable

PET: Positron emission tomography

RBC: Red blood cell

ROS: Reactive oxygen species, also called free radical

SOD: Superoxide dismutase

TBARS: Thiobarbituric acid reactive substances

TBI: Traumatic brain injury

TNF-alpha: Tumor necrosis factor-alpha

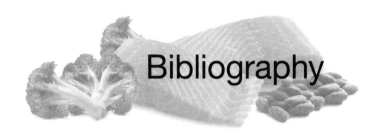

Bibliography

"1994–2004, The Development of DRI's." 2008. Lessons Learned and New Challenges: Workshop. Washington D.C.: National Academic Press.

Aarsland, D., A. Rongve, S. P. Nore, et al. 2008. Frequency and case identification of dementia with Lewy bodies using the revised consensus criteria. *Dement Geriatr Cogn Disord* 26, no. 5: 445–52.

Abate, A., G. Yang, P. A. Dennery, et al. 2000. Synergistic inhibition of cyclo-oxygenase-2 expression by vitamin E and aspirin. *Free Radic Biol Med* 29, no. 11: 1135–42.

Al Moutaery, K., S. Al Deeb, H. Ahmad Khan, et al. 2003. Caffeine impairs short-term neurological outcome after concussive head injury in rats. *Neurosurgery* 53, no. 3: 704–11.

Albanes, D., O. P. Heinonen, J. K. Huttunen, et al. 1995. Effects of alpha-tocopherol and beta-carotene supplements on cancer incidence in the Alpha-Tocopherol Beta-Carotene Cancer Prevention Study. *Am J Clin Nutr* 62, no. 6 Suppl: 1427S–1430S.

Ansari, M. A., K. N. Roberts, and S. W. Scheff. 2008. Oxidative stress and modification of synaptic proteins in hippocampus after traumatic brain injury. *Free Radic Biol Med* 45, no. 4: 443–52.

Asmus, K. D., and M. Bonifacic. 1994. "Free radical chemistry." In: *Excercise and Oxygen Toxicity.* Edited by C. K. Sen, L. Packer, and O. Hanninen. New York: Elsevier.

Ates, O., S. Cayli, E. Altinoz, et al. 2007. Neuroprotection by resveratrol against traumatic brain injury in rats. *Mol Cell Biochem* 294, nos. 1–2: 137–44.

Aygok, G. A., A. Marmarou, P. Fatouros, et al. 2008. Assessment of mitochondrial impairment and cerebral blood flow in severe brain injured patients. *Acta Neurochir Suppl* 102: 57–61.

Baldacara, L., A. P. Jackowski, A. Schoedl, et al. 2011. Reduced cerebellar left hemisphere and vermal volume in adults with PTSD from a community sample. *J Psychiatr Res* 45, no. 12: 1627–33.

Barger, S. W., M. E. Goodwin, M. M. Porter, et al. 2007. Glutamate release from activated microglia requires the oxidative burst and lipid peroxidation. *J Neurochem* 101, no. 5: 1205–13.

Baum, M. K., A. Campa, S. Lai, et al. 2013. Effect of micronutrient supplementation on disease progression in asymptomatic, antiretroviral-naive, HIV-infected adults in Botswana: a randomized clinical trial. *JAMA* 310, no. 20: 2154–63.

Bayir, H., P. D. Adelson, S. R. Wisniewski, et al. 2009. Therapeutic hypothermia preserves antioxidant defenses after severe traumatic brain injury in infants and children. *Crit Care Med* 37, no. 2: 689–95.

Bayir, H., V. E. Kagan, Y. Y. Tyurina, et al. 2002. Assessment of antioxidant reserves and oxidative stress in cerebrospinal fluid after severe traumatic brain injury in infants and children. *Pediatr Res* 51, no. 5: 571–78.

Bayir, H., P. M. Kochanek, and V. E. Kagan. 2006. Oxidative stress in immature brain after traumatic brain injury. *Dev Neurosci* 28, nos. 4–5: 420–31.

Belli, A., J. Sen, A. Petzold, et al. 2006. Extracellular N-acetylaspartate depletion in traumatic brain injury. *J Neurochem* 96, no. 3: 861–69.

Beni, S. M., R. Kohen, R. J. Reiter, et al. 2004. Melatonin-induced neuroprotection after closed head injury is associated with increased brain antioxidants and attenuated late-phase activation of NF-kappaB and AP-1. *FASEB J* 18, no. 1: 149–51.

Bergstrom, P., H. C. Andersson, Y. Gao, et al. 2011. Repeated transient sulforaphane stimulation in astrocytes leads to prolonged Nrf2-mediated gene expression and protection from superoxide-induced damage. *Neuropharmacology* 60, nos. 2–3: 343–53.

Bermpohl, D., Z. You, E. H. Lo, et al. 2007. TNF alpha and Fas mediate tissue damage and functional outcome after traumatic brain injury in mice. *J Cereb Blood Flow Metab* 27, no. 11: 1806–18.

Beschorner, R., T. D. Nguyen, F. Gozalan, et al. 2002. CD14 expression by activated parenchymal microglia/macrophages and infiltrating monocytes following human traumatic brain injury. *Acta Neuropathol* 103, no. 6: 541–49.

Breedlove, E. L., M. Robinson, T. M. Talavage, et al. 2012. Biomechanical correlates of symptomatic and asymptomatic neurophysiological impairment in high school football. *J Biomech* 45, no. 7: 1265–72.

Bremner, J. D. 2006. Stress and brain atrophy. *CNS Neurol Disord Drug Targets* 5, no. 5: 503–12.

Bremner, J. D., J. Licinio, A. Darnell, et al. 1997. Elevated CSF corticotropin-releasing factor concentrations in posttraumatic stress disorder. *Am J Psychiatry* 154, no. 5: 624–29.

Bremner, J. D., T. M. Scott, R. C. Delaney, et al. 1993. Deficits in short-term memory in posttraumatic stress disorder. *Am J Psychiatry* 150, no. 7: 1015–19.

Bullock, R., A. Zauner, J. J. Woodward, et al. 1998. Factors affecting excitatory amino acid release following severe human head injury. *J Neurosurg* 89, no. 4: 507–18.

Burriss, L., E. Ayers, J. Ginsberg, et al. 2008. Learning and memory impairment in PTSD: relationship to depression. *Depress Anxiety* 25, no. 2: 149–57.

Butterfield, D. A. 2002. Amyloid beta-peptide (1-42)-induced oxidative stress and neurotoxicity: implications for neurodegeneration in Alzheimer's disease brain. A review. *Free Radic Res* 36, no. 12: 1307–13.

Buttram, S. D., S. R. Wisniewski, E. K. Jackson, et al. 2007. Multiplex assessment of cytokine and chemokine levels in cerebrospinal fluid following severe pediatric traumatic brain injury: effects of moderate hypothermia. *J Neurotrauma* 24, no. 11: 1707–17.

Cardenas, V. A., K. Samuelson, M. Lenoci, et al. 2011. Changes in brain anatomy during the course of posttraumatic stress disorder. *Psychiatry Res* 193, no. 2: 93–100.

Carlson, K. F., S. M. Kehle, L. A. Meis, et al. 2011. Prevalence, assessment, and treatment of mild traumatic brain injury and posttraumatic stress disorder: a systematic review of the evidence. *J Head Trauma Rehabil* 26, no. 2: 103–15.

Casson, I. R., D. C. Viano, J. W. Powell, et al. 2011. Repeat concussions in the national football league. *Sports Health* 3, no. 1: 11–24.

Castro, C. A., and C. W. Hoge. 2005. "Building psychological resiliency and mitigating the risks of combat and deployment stressors faced by soldiers."

Presented at NATO Human Factors and Medicine Panel Symposium, Prague, Czech Republic, October 3–5, 2005.

Chamoun, R., D. Suki, S. P. Gopinath, et al. 2010. Role of extracellular glutamate measured by cerebral microdialysis in severe traumatic brain injury. *J Neurosurg* 113, no. 3: 564–70.

Chan, K., X. D. Han, and Y. W. Kan. 2001. An important function of Nrf2 in combating oxidative stress: detoxification of acetaminophen. *Proc Natl Acad Sci U S A* 98, no. 8: 4611–16.

Chen, G., Q. Fang, J. Zhang, et al. 2011. Role of the Nrf2-ARE pathway in early brain injury after experimental subarachnoid hemorrhage. *J Neurosci Res* 89, no. 4: 515–23.

Chen, G., J. Shi, Z. Hu, et al. 2008. Inhibitory effect on cerebral inflammatory response following traumatic brain injury in rats: a potential neuroprotective mechanism of n-acetylcysteine. *Mediators Inflamm* 2008:716458.

Chen, R.S., C. C. Huang, and N.S. Chu. 1997. Coenzyme Q10 treatment in mitochondrial encephalomyopathies. Short-term double-blind, crossover study. *Eur Neurol* 37: 212–18.

Chen, X. R., V. C. Besson, B. Palmier, et al. 2007. Neurological recovery-promoting, anti-inflammatory, and anti-oxidative effects afforded by fenofibrate, a PPAR alpha agonist, in traumatic brain injury. *J Neurotrauma* 24, no. 7: 1119–31.

Chen, X., I. Y. Choi, T. S. Chang, et al. 2009. Pretreatment with interferon-gamma protects microglia from oxidative stress via up-regulation of Mn-SOD. *Free Radic Biol Med* 46, no. 8: 1204–10.

Chinta, S. J., and J. K. Andersen. 2005. Dopaminergic neurons. *Int J Biochem Cell Biol* 37, no. 5: 942–46.

Choi, H. K., Y. R. Pokharel, S. C. Lim, et al. 2009. Inhibition of liver fibrosis by solubilized coenzyme Q10: Role of Nrf2 activation in inhibiting transforming growth factor-beta1 expression. *Toxicol Appl Pharmacol* 240, no. 3: 377–84.

Clausen, F., A. Hanell, M. Bjork, et al. 2009. Neutralization of interleukin-1beta modifies the inflammatory response and improves histological and cognitive outcome following traumatic brain injury in mice. *Eur J Neurosci* 30, no. 3: 385–96.

Clausen, F., N. Marklund, A. Lewen, et al. 2012. Interstitial F(2)-isoprostane

8-iso-PGF(2alpha) as a biomarker of oxidative stress after severe human traumatic brain injury. *J Neurotrauma* 29, no. 5: 766–75.

Conley, Y. P., D. O. Okonkwo, S. Deslouches, et al. 2013. Mitochondrial polymorphisms impact outcomes after severe traumatic brain injury. *J Neurotrauma* 31, no. 1: 34–41.

Conte, V., K. Uryu, S. Fujimoto, et al. 2004. Vitamin E reduces amyloidosis and improves cognitive function in Tg2576 mice following repetitive concussive brain injury. *J Neurochem* 90, no. 3: 758–64.

Cotran, R. S., V. Kumar, and T. Collins, ed. 1999. *Disease of Immunity, Pathologic Basis of Disease*. New York: W. B. Saunders Company.

Covassin, T., P. Schatz, and C. B. Swanik. 2007. Sex differences in neuropsychological function and post-concussion symptoms of concussed collegiate athletes. *Neurosurgery* 61, no. 2: 345–50.

Dai, S. S., Y. G. Zhou, W. Li, et al. 2010. Local glutamate level dictates adenosine A2A receptor regulation of neuroinflammation and traumatic brain injury. *J Neurosci* 30, no. 16: 5802–10.

Darwish, R. S., and N. S. Amiridze. 2010. Detectable levels of cytochrome C and activated caspase-9 in cerebrospinal fluid after human traumatic brain injury. *Neurocrit Care* 12, no. 3: 337–41.

Darwish, R. S., N. Amiridze, and B. Aarabi. 2007. Nitrotyrosine as an oxidative stress marker: evidence for involvement in neurologic outcome in human traumatic brain injury. *J Trauma* 63, no. 2: 439–42.

Dash, P. K., S. A. Orsi, M. Zhang, et al. 2010. Valproate administered after traumatic brain injury provides neuroprotection and improves cognitive function in rats. *PLoS One* 5, no. 6: e11383.

Davis, M., K. Ressler, B. O. Rothbaum, et al. 2006. Effects of D-cycloserine on extinction: translation from preclinical to clinical work. *Biol Psychiatry* 60, no. 4: 369–75.

De Beaumont, L., S. Tremblay, J. Poirier, et al. 2012. Altered bidirectional plasticity and reduced implicit motor learning in concussed athletes. *Cereb Cortex* 22, no. 1: 112–21.

de Quervain, D. J., and J. Margraf. 2008. Glucocorticoids for the treatment of post-traumatic stress disorder and phobias: a novel therapeutic approach. *Eur J Pharmacol* 583, nos. 2–3: 365–71.

Devaraj, S., R. Tang, B. Adams-Huet, et al. 2007. Effect of high-dose alpha-tocopherol supplementation on biomarkers of oxidative stress and inflammation and carotid atherosclerosis in patients with coronary artery disease. *Am J Clin Nutr* 86, no. 5: 1392–98.

Diehl, L. A., L. O. Alvares, C. Noschang, et al. 2012. Long-lasting effects of maternal separation on an animal model of post-traumatic stress disorder: effects on memory and hippocampal oxidative stress. *Neurochem Res* 37, no. 4: 700–707.

Dohi, K., K. Satoh, Y. Mihara, et al. 2006. Alkoxyl radical-scavenging activity of edaravone in patients with traumatic brain injury. *J Neurotrauma* 23, no. 11: 1591–99.

Ellemberg, D., L. C. Henry, S. N. Macciocchi, et al. 2009. Advances in sport concussion assessment: from behavioral to brain imaging measures. *J Neurotrauma* 26, no. 12: 2365–82.

Emmerling, M. R., M. C. Morganti-Kossmann, T. Kossmann, et al. 2000. Traumatic brain injury elevates the Alzheimer's amyloid peptide A beta 42 in human CSF. A possible role for nerve cell injury. *Ann N Y Acad Sci* 903: 118–22.

Erickson, J. T., T. A. Brosenitsch, and D. M. Katz. 2001. Brain-derived neurotrophic factor and glial cell line-derived neurotrophic factor are required simultaneously for survival of dopaminergic primary sensory neurons in vivo. *J Neurosci* 21, no. 2: 581–89.

Fang, W. H., D. L. Wang, and F. Wang. 2006. [Expression of c-myc protein on rats' brains after brain concussion]. *Fa Yi Xue Za Zhi* 22, no. 5: 333–34.

Farina, N., M. G. Isaac, A. R. Clark, et al. 2012. Vitamin E for Alzheimer's dementia and mild cognitive impairment. *Cochrane Database Syst Rev* 11: CD002854.

Fleming, J. T., W. He, C. Hao, et al. 2013. The Purkinje neuron acts as a central regulator of spatially and functionally distinct cerebellar precursors. *Dev Cell* 27, no. 3: 278–92.

Foley, K., R. E. Kast, and E. L. Altschuler. 2009. Ritonavir and disulfiram have potential to inhibit caspase-1 mediated inflammation and reduce neurological sequelae after minor blast exposure. *Med Hypotheses* 72, no. 2: 150–52.

Fox, J. L., E. N. Vu, M. Doyle-Waters, et al. 2010. Prophylactic hypothermia for traumatic brain injury: a quantitative systematic review. *CJEM* 12, no. 4: 355–64.

Friedman, M. J. 2005. Veterans' mental health in the wake of war. *N Engl J Med* 352, no. 13: 1287–90.

Frugier, T., M. C. Morganti-Kossmann, D. O'Reilly, et al. 2010. In situ detection of inflammatory mediators in post mortem human brain tissue after traumatic injury. *J Neurotrauma* 27, no. 3: 497–507.

Fu, Y., S. Zheng, J. Lin, et al. 2008. Curcumin protects the rat liver from CCl4-caused injury and fibrogenesis by attenuating oxidative stress and suppressing inflammation. *Mol Pharmacol* 73, no. 2: 399–409.

Gahm, C., S. Holmin, and T. Mathiesen. 2002. Nitric oxide synthase expression after human brain contusion. *Neurosurgery* 50, no. 6: 1319–26.

Gahm, C., S. Holmin, P. N. Wiklund, et al. 2006. Neuroprotection by selective inhibition of inducible nitric oxide synthase after experimental brain contusion. *J Neurotrauma* 23, no. 9: 1343–54.

Gao, L., J. Wang, K. R. Sekhar, et al. 2007. Novel n-3 fatty acid oxidation products activate Nrf2 by destabilizing the association between Keap1 and Cullin3. *J Biol Chem* 282, no. 4: 2529–37.

Gaziano, J. M., H. D. Sesso, W. G. Christen, et al. 2012. Multivitamins in the prevention of cancer in men: the Physicians' Health Study II randomized controlled trial. *JAMA* 308, no. 18: 1871–80.

Gessel, L. M., S. K. Fields, C. L. Collins, et al. 2007. Concussions among United States high school and collegiate athletes. *J Athl Train* 42, no. 4: 495–503.

Gilmer, L. K., K. N. Roberts, K. Joy, et al. 2009. Early mitochondrial dysfunction after cortical contusion injury. *J Neurotrauma* 26, no. 8: 1271–80.

Globus, M. Y., O. Alonso, W. D. Dietrich, et al. 1995. Glutamate release and free radical production following brain injury: effects of posttraumatic hypothermia. *J Neurochem* 65, no. 4: 1704–11.

Gola, H., H. Engler, A. Sommershof, et al. 2013. Posttraumatic stress disorder is associated with an enhanced spontaneous production of pro-inflammatory cytokines by peripheral blood mononuclear cells. *BMC Psychiatry* 13: 40.

Goodman, J. C., M. Van, S. P. Gopinath, et al. 2008. Pro-inflammatory and pro-apoptotic elements of the neuroinflammatory response are activated in traumatic brain injury. *Acta Neurochir Suppl* 102: 437–39.

Goodrich, G. S., A. Y. Kabakov, M. Q. Hameed, et al. 2013. Ceftriaxone treatment after traumatic brain injury restores expression of the glutamate transporter, GLT-1, reduces regional gliosis, and reduces post-traumatic seizures in the rat. *J Neurotrauma* 30, no. 16: 1434–41.

Gopinath, S. P., A. B. Valadka, J. C. Goodman, et al. 2000. Extracellular glutamate and aspartate in head injured patients. *Acta Neurochir Suppl* 76: 437–38.

Gottshall, K., A. Drake, N. Gray, et al. 2003. Objective vestibular tests as outcome measures in head injury patients. *Laryngoscope* 113, no. 10: 1746–50.

Gottshall, K. R., M. E. Hoffer, B. J. Balough. June, 2006. "Use of antioxidants micronutrient compounds in vestibular rehabilitation after operational head trauma or blast injury." Paper read at Barany International Balance Meeting, at Stockholm, Sweden.

Gradus, J. L. 2011. Epidemiology of PTSD. *National Center for PTSD*.

Grasso, G., A. Sfacteria, F. Meli, et al. 2007. Neuroprotection by erythropoietin administration after experimental traumatic brain injury. *Brain Res* 1182: 99–105.

Green, K. N., J. S. Steffan, H. Martinez-Coria, et al. 2008. Nicotinamide restores cognition in Alzheimer's disease transgenic mice via a mechanism involving sirtuin inhibition and selective reduction of Thr231-phosphotau. *J Neurosci* 28, no. 45: 11500–10.

Guo, M., T. Liu, J. C. Guo, et al. 2012. Study on serum cytokine levels in post-traumatic stress disorder patients. *Asian Pac J Trop Med* 5, no. 4: 323–25.

Guskiewicz, K. M., S. W. Marshall, J. Bailes, et al. 2005. Association between recurrent concussion and late-life cognitive impairment in retired professional football players. *Neurosurgery* 57, no. 4: 719–26.

Guskiewicz, K. M., M. McCrea, S. W. Marshall, et al. 2003. Cumulative effects associated with recurrent concussion in collegiate football players: the NCAA Concussion Study. *JAMA* 290, no. 19: 2549–55.

Guskiewicz, K. M., N. L. Weaver, D. A. Padua, et al. 2000. Epidemiology of concussion in collegiate and high school football players. *Am J Sports Med* 28, no. 5: 643–50.

Hakan, T., H. Z. Toklu, N. Biber, et al. 2009. Effect of COX-2 inhibitor meloxicam against traumatic brain injury-induced biochemical, histopathological changes and blood-brain barrier permeability. *Neurol Res* 32, no. 6: 629–35.

Hall, E. D., M. R. Detloff, K. Johnson, et al. 2004. Peroxynitrite-mediated protein nitration and lipid peroxidation in a mouse model of traumatic brain injury. *J Neurotrauma* 21, no. 1: 9–20.

Halterman, C. I., J. Langan, A. Drew, et al. 2006. Tracking the recovery of visuospatial attention deficits in mild traumatic brain injury. *Brain* 129, Pt 3: 747–53.

Hamner, M. B., S. Robert, and B. C. Frueh. 2004. Treatment-resistant post-traumatic stress disorder: strategies for intervention. *CNS Spectr* 9, no. 10: 740–52.

Hang, C. H., G. Chen, J. X. Shi, et al. 2006. Cortical expression of nuclear factor kappaB after human brain contusion. *Brain Res* 1109, no. 1: 14–21.

Harvey, B. H., T. Bothma, A. Nel, et al. 2005. Involvement of the NMDA receptor, NO-cyclic GMP and nuclear factor K-beta in an animal model of repeated trauma. *Hum Psychopharmacol* 20, no. 5: 367–73.

Harvey, B. H., F. Oosthuizen, L. Brand, et al. 2004. Stress-restress evokes sustained iNOS activity and altered GABA levels and NMDA receptors in rat hippocampus. *Psychopharmacology (Berl)* 175, no. 4: 494–502.

Hascup, E. R., K. N. Hascup, M. Stephens, et al. 2010. Rapid microelectrode measurements and the origin and regulation of extracellular glutamate in rat prefrontal cortex. *J Neurochem* 115, no. 6: 1608–20.

Hausmann, R., A. Kaiser, C. Lang, et al. 1999. A quantitative immunohisto-chemical study on the time-dependent course of acute inflammatory cellular response to human brain injury. *Int J Legal Med* 112, no. 4: 227–32.

Hayes, J. D., S. A. Chanas, C. J. Henderson, et al. 2000. The Nrf2 transcription factor contributes both to the basal expression of glutathione S-transferases in mouse liver and to their induction by the chemopreventive synthetic antioxidants, butylated hydroxyanisole and ethoxyquin. *Biochem Soc Trans* 28, no. 2: 33–41.

Hein, A. M., and M. K. O'Banion. 2009. Neuroinflammation and memory: the role of prostaglandins. *Mol Neurobiol* 40, no. 1: 15–32.

Hennekens, C. H., J. E. Buring, J. E. Manson, et al. 1996. Lack of effect of long-term supplementation with beta-carotene on the incidence of malignant neoplasm and cardiovascular disease. *N Eng J Med* 334: 1145–49.

Heresco-Levy, U., A. Vass, B. Bloch, et al. 2009. Pilot controlled trial of D-serine for the treatment of post-traumatic stress disorder. *Int J Neuropsychopharmacol* 12, no. 9: 1275–82.

Hicks, R. R., S. J. Fertig, R. E. Desrocher, et al. 2010. Neurological effects of blast injury. *J Trauma* 68, no. 5: 1257–63.

Hine, C. M., and J. R. Mitchell. 2012. NRF2 and the Phase II Response in Acute Stress Resistance Induced by Dietary Restriction. *J Clin Exp Pathol* S4, no. 4.

Hinzman, J. M., T. C. Thomas, J. E. Quintero, et al. 2012. Disruptions in the regulation of extracellular glutamate by neurons and glia in the rat striatum two days after diffuse brain injury. *J Neurotrauma* 29, no. 6: 1197–208.

Hoge, C. W., C. A. Castro, S. C. Messer, et al. 2004. Combat duty in Iraq and Afghanistan, mental health problems, and barriers to care. *N Engl J Med* 351, no. 1: 13–22.

Hoge, C. W., D. McGurk, J. L. Thomas, et al. 2008. Mild traumatic brain injury in U.S. Soldiers returning from Iraq. *N Engl J Med* 358, no. 5: 453–63.

Hoge, E. A., K. Brandstetter, S. Moshier, et al. 2009. Broad spectrum of cytokine abnormalities in panic disorder and posttraumatic stress disorder. *Depress Anxiety* 26, no. 5: 447–55.

Hohl, A., S. Gullo Jda, C. C. Silva, et al. 2012. Plasma levels of oxidative stress biomarkers and hospital mortality in severe head injury: a multivariate analysis. *J Crit Care* 27, no. 5: 523 e11-9.

Holland, E. C., and H. E. Varmus. 1998. Basic fibroblast growth factor induces cell migration and proliferation after glia-specific gene transfer in mice. *Proc Natl Acad Sci USA* 95, no. 3: 1218–23.

Holmin, S., and B. Hojeberg. 2004. In situ detection of intracerebral cytokine expression after human brain contusion. *Neurosci Lett* 369, no. 2: 108–14.

Holmin, S., J. Soderlund, P. Biberfeld, et al. 1998. Intracerebral inflammation after human brain contusion. *Neurosurgery* 42, no. 2: 291–98.

Holtmeier, W., and D. Kabelitz. 2005. Gammadelta T cells link innate and adaptive immune responses. *Chem Immunol Allergy* 86: 151–83.

Houlgatte, R., M. Mallat, P. Brachet, et al. 1989. Secretion of nerve growth factor in cultures of glial cells and neurons derived from different regions of the mouse brain. *J Neurosci Res* 24, no. 2: 143–52.

Hutchinson, P. J., M. T. O'Connell, N. J. Rothwell, et al. 2007. Inflammation in human brain injury: intracerebral concentrations of IL-1alpha, IL-1beta, and their endogenous inhibitor IL-1ra. *J Neurotrauma* 24, no. 10: 1545–57.

Huttemann, M., I. Lee, C. W. Kreipke, et al. 2008. Suppression of the inducible form of nitric oxide synthase prior to traumatic brain injury improves cytochrome c oxidase activity and normalizes cellular energy levels. *Neuroscience* 151, no. 1: 148–54.

Ipser, J., S. Seedat, and D. J. Stein. 2006. Pharmacotherapy for post-traumatic stress disorder—a systematic review and meta-analysis. *S Afr Med J* 96, no. 10: 1088–96.

Itoh, K., T. Chiba, S. Takahashi, et al. 1997. An Nrf2/small Maf heterodimer mediates the induction of phase II detoxifying enzyme genes through antioxidant response elements. *Biochem Biophys Res Commun* 236, no. 2: 313–22.

Ji, L., R. Liu, X. D. Zhang, et al. 2010. N-acetylcysteine attenuates phosgene-induced acute lung injury via up-regulation of Nrf2 expression. *Inhal Toxicol* 22, no. 7: 535–42.

Jin, W., H. Wang, W. Yan, et al. 2008. Disruption of Nrf2 enhances upregulation of nuclear factor-kappaB activity, proinflammatory cytokines, and intercellular adhesion molecule-1 in the brain after traumatic brain injury. *Mediators Inflamm* 2008:725174.

Jin, W., H. Wang, W. Yan, et al. 2009. Role of Nrf2 in protection against traumatic brain injury in mice. *J Neurotrauma* 26, no. 1: 131–39.

Kanninen, K., T. M. Malm, H. K. Jyrkkanen, et al. 2008. Nuclear factor erythroid 2-related factor 2 protects against beta amyloid. *Mol Cell Neurosci* 39, no. 3: 302–13.

Kasai, K., H. Yamasue, M. W. Gilbertson, et al. 2008. Evidence for acquired pregenual anterior cingulate gray matter loss from a twin study of combat-related posttraumatic stress disorder. *Biol Psychiatry* 63, no. 6: 550–56.

Kehrer, J. P., and C. V. Smith. 1994. "Free radicals in biology: sources, reactivities, and roles in the etiology of human diseases." In: *Natural Antioxidants in Human Health and Disease.* Edited by B. Frei. New York: Academy Press, Inc.

Kehry, M. R., and P. D. Hodgkin. 1994. B-cell activation by helper T-cell membranes. *Crit Rev Immunol* 14, nos. 3–4: 221–38.

Kerr, Z. Y., S. W. Marshall, H. P. Harding, Jr, et al. 2012. Nine-year risk of depression diagnosis increases with increasing self-reported concussions in retired professional football players. *Am J Sports Med* 40, no. 10: 2206–12.

Kessler, R. C., W. T. Chiu, O. Demler, et al. 2005. Prevalence, severity, and comorbidity of 12-month DSM-IV disorders in the National Comorbidity Survey Replication. *Arch Gen Psychiatry* 62, no. 6: 617–27.

Khan, M., Y. B. Im, A. Shunmugavel, et al. 2009. Administration of S-nitrosoglutathione after traumatic brain injury protects the neurovascular unit and reduces secondary injury in a rat model of controlled cortical impact. *J Neuroinflammation* 6: 32.

King, D. W., G. A. Leskin, and F. W. Weathers. 1998. Confirmatory factor analysis of the clinician-administered PTSD scale: Evidence for the dimensionality of postraumatic stress disorder. *Psychological Assessment* 10: 90–96.

King, J., V. Mackey, K. Prasad, et al. April, 2008. Blockage of the proposed precipitating stage for Parkinson's disease by antioxidants: a potential preventive measure for PD. Paper read at FASEB, at San Diego.

Kode, A., S. Rajendrasozhan, S. Caito, et al. 2008. Resveratrol induces glutathione synthesis by activation of Nrf2 and protects against cigarette smoke-mediated oxidative stress in human lung epithelial cells. *Am J Physiol Lung Cell Mol Physiol* 294, no. 3: L478–88.

Koura, S. S., E. M. Doppenberg, A. Marmarou, et al. 1998. Relationship between excitatory amino acid release and outcome after severe human head injury. *Acta Neurochir Suppl* 71: 244–46.

Kuhn, S., and J. Gallinat. 2013. Gray matter correlates of posttraumatic stress disorder: a quantitative meta-analysis. *Biol Psychiatry* 73, no. 1: 70–74.

Langermans, J. A., W. L. Hazenbos, and R. van Furth. 1994. Antimicrobial functions of mononuclear phagocytes. *J Immunol Methods* 174, nos. 1–2: 185–94.

Lee, H. S., K. K. Jung, J. Y. Cho, et al. 2007. Neuroprotective effect of curcumin is mainly mediated by blockade of microglial cell activation. *Pharmazie* 62, no. 12: 937–42.

Lee, T. M., M. L. Wong, B. W. Lau, et al. 2014. Aerobic exercise interacts with neurotrophic factors to predict cognitive functioning in adolescents. *Psychoneuroendocrinology* 39: 214–24.

Leppala, J. M., J. Virtamo, and R. Fogelholm. 2000. Controlled trial of alphatocopherol and beta-carotene supplements on stroke incidence and mortality in male smokers. *Arterioscler Thromb Vasc Biol* 20, no. 1: 230–35.

Leung, L. Y., G. Wei, D. A. Shear, et al. 2013. The acute effects of hemorrhagic shock on cerebral blood flow, brain tissue oxygen tension, and spreading depolarization following penetrating ballistic-like brain injury. *J Neurotrauma* 30, no. 14: 1288–98.

Levy, M. L., B. M. Ozgur, C. Berry, et al. 2004. Analysis and evolution of head injury in football. *Neurosurgery* 55, no. 3: 649–55.

Li, X. H., C. Y. Li, J. M. Lu, et al. 2012. Allicin ameliorates cognitive deficits ageing-induced learning and memory deficits through enhancing of Nrf2 antioxidant signaling pathways. *Neurosci Lett* 514, no. 1: 46–50.

Lima, F. D., M. A. Souza, A. F. Furian, et al. 2008. Na+,K+-ATPase activity impairment after experimental traumatic brain injury: relationship to spatial learning deficits and oxidative stress. *Behav Brain Res* 193, no. 2: 306–10.

Lin, Y., and L. Wen. 2013. Inflammatory response following diffuse axonal injury. *Int J Med Sci* 10, no. 5: 515–21.

Lincoln, A. E., S. V. Caswell, J. L. Almquist, et al. 2011. Trends in concussion incidence in high school sports: a prospective 11-year study. *Am J Sports Med* 39, no. 5: 958–63.

Litman, G. W., J. P. Cannon, and L. J. Dishaw. 2005. Reconstructing immune phylogeny: new perspectives. *Nat Rev Immunol* 5, no. 11: 866–79.

Liu, D., M. Pitta, and M. P. Mattson. 2008. Preventing NAD(+) depletion protects neurons against excitotoxicity: bioenergetic effects of mild mitochondrial uncoupling and caloric restriction. *Ann N Y Acad Sci* 1147: 275–82.

Lloyd, E., K. Somera-Molina, L. J. Van Eldik, et al. 2008. Suppression of acute proinflammatory cytokine and chemokine upregulation by post-injury administration of a novel small molecule improves long-term neurologic outcome in a mouse model of traumatic brain injury. *J Neuroinflammation* 5: 28.

Louin, G., C. Marchand-Verrecchia, B. Palmier, et al. 2006. Selective inhibition of inducible nitric oxide synthase reduces neurological deficit but not cerebral edema following traumatic brain injury. *Neuropharmacology* 50, no. 2: 182–90.

MacGregor, A. J., A. L. Dougherty, R. H. Morrison, et al. 2011. Repeated concussion among U.S. military personnel during Operation Iraqi Freedom. *J Rehabil Res Dev* 48, no. 10: 1269–78.

Maes, M., A. H. Lin, L. Delmeire, et al. 1999. Elevated serum interleukin-6 (IL-6) and IL-6 receptor concentrations in posttraumatic stress disorder following accidental man-made traumatic events. *Biol Psychiatry* 45, no. 7: 833–39.

Maier, B., M. Lehnert, H. L. Laurer, et al. 2006. Delayed elevation of soluble tumor necrosis factor receptors p75 and p55 in cerebrospinal fluid and plasma after traumatic brain injury. *Shock* 26, no. 2: 122–27.

Martin, P., and S. J. Leibovich. 2005. Inflammatory cells during wound repair: the good, the bad and the ugly. *Trends Cell Biol* 15, no. 11: 599–607.

Matsuoka, Y., D. Nishi, N. Nakaya, et al. 2011. Attenuating posttraumatic distress with omega-3 polyunsaturated fatty acids among disaster medical assistance team members after the Great East Japan Earthquake: the APOP randomized controlled trial. *BMC Psychiatry* 11: 132.

Matzinger, P. 2002. The danger model: a renewed sense of self. *Science* 296 (5566): 301–5.

Mazzeo, A. T., A. Beat, A. Singh, et al. 2009. The role of mitochondrial transition pore, and its modulation, in traumatic brain injury and delayed neurodegeneration after TBI. *Exp Neurol* 218, no. 2: 363–70.

Medzhitov, R. 2007. Recognition of microorganisms and activation of the immune response. *Nature* 449, no. 7164: 819–26.

Melamed, S., A. Shirom, S. Toker, et al. 2004. Association of fear of terror with low-grade inflammation among apparently healthy employed adults. *Psychosom Med* 66, no. 4: 484–91.

Mellergard, P., F. Sjogren, and J. Hillman. 2012. The cerebral extracellular release of glycerol, glutamate, and FGF2 is increased in older patients following severe traumatic brain injury. *J Neurotrauma* 29, no. 1: 112–18.

Mikawa, S., H. Kinouchi, H. Kamii, et al. 1996. Attenuation of acute and chronic damage following traumatic brain injury in copper, zinc-superoxide dismutase transgenic mice. *J Neurosurg* 85, no. 5: 885–91.

Miller, R. J., A. G. Sutherland, J. D. Hutchison, et al. 2001. C-reactive protein and interleukin 6 receptor in post-traumatic stress disorder: a pilot study. *Cytokine* 13, no. 4: 253–55.

Minambres, E., A. Cemborian, P. Sanchez-Velasco, et al. 2003. Correlation between transcranial interleukin-6 gradient and outcome in patients with acute brain injury. *Crit. Care Med.* 31: 33–38.

Murrough, J. W., Y. Huang, J. Hu, et al. 2011. Reduced amygdala serotonin transporter binding in posttraumatic stress disorder. *Biol Psychiatry* 70, no. 11: 1033–38.

Mustafa, A. G., I. N. Singh, J. Wang, et al. 2010. Mitochondrial protection after traumatic brain injury by scavenging lipid peroxyl radicals. *J Neurochem* 114, no. 1: 271–80.

Nair, J., and S. Singh Ajit. 2008. The role of the glutamatergic system in posttraumatic stress disorder. *CNS Spectr* 13, no. 7: 585–91.

Nayak, C. D., D. M. Nayak, A. Raja, et al. 2008. Erythrocyte indicators of oxidative changes in patients with graded traumatic head injury. *Neurol India* 56, no. 1: 31–35.

Niture, S. K., J. W. Kaspar, J. Shen, et al. 2010. Nrf2 signaling and cell survival. *Toxicol Appl Pharmacol* 244, no. 1: 37–42.

Opii, W. O., V. N. Nukala, R. Sultana, et al. 2007. Proteomic identification of oxidized mitochondrial proteins following experimental traumatic brain injury. *J Neurotrauma* 24, no. 5: 772–89.

Pall, M. L., and J. D. Satterlee. 2001. Elevated nitric oxide/peroxynitrite mechanism for the common etiology of multiple chemical sensitivity, chronic fatigue syndrome, and posttraumatic stress disorder. *Ann N Y Acad Sci* 933: 323–29.

Pandya, J. D., J. R. Pauly, V. N. Nukala, et al. 2007. Post-Injury Administration of Mitochondrial Uncouplers Increases Tissue Sparing and Improves Behavioral Outcome following Traumatic Brain Injury in Rodents. *J Neurotrauma* 24, no. 5: 798–811.

Panter, S. S., and A. I. Faden. 1992. Pretreatment with NMDA antagonists limits release of excitatory amino acids following traumatic brain injury. *Neurosci Lett* 136, no. 2: 165–68.

Pappolla, M. A., Y. J. Chyan, R. A. Omar, et al. 1998. Evidence of oxidative stress and in vivo neurotoxicity of beta-amyloid in a transgenic mouse model of Alzheimer's disease: a chronic oxidative paradigm for testing antioxidant therapies in vivo. *Am J Pathol* 152, no. 4: 871–77.

Peairs, A. T., and J. W. Rankin. 2008. Inflammatory response to a high-fat, low-carbohydrate weight loss diet: Effect of antioxidants. *Obesity (Silver Spring)* 16, no. 7: 1573–78.

Petronilho, F., G. Feier, B. de Souza, et al. 2009. Oxidative stress in brain according to traumatic brain injury intensity. *J Surg Res* 164, no. 2: 316–20.

Pivac, N., J. Knezevic, D. Kozaric-Kovacic, et al. 2007. Monoamine oxidase (MAO) intron 13 polymorphism and platelet MAO-B activity in combat-related posttraumatic stress disorder. *J Affect Disord* 103, nos. 1–3: 131–38.

Potts, M. B., S. E. Koh, W. D. Whetstone, et al. 2006. Traumatic injury to the immature brain: inflammation, oxidative injury, and iron-mediated damage as potential therapeutic targets. *NeuroRx* 3, no. 2: 143–53.

Prasad, K. N., R. J. Cohrs, and O. K. Sharma. 1990. Decreased expressions of c-myc and H-ras oncogenes in vitamin E succinate induced morphologically differentiated murine B-16 melanoma cells in culture. *Biochem Cell Biol* 68, no. 11: 1250–55.

Prasad, K. N., W. C. Cole, and K. C. Prasad. 2002. Risk factors for Alzheimer's disease: role of multiple antioxidants, non-steroidal anti-inflammatory and cholinergic agents alone or in combination in prevention and treatment. *J Am Coll Nutr* 21, no. 6: 506–22.

Prasad, K. N. 2011. *Micronutrients in Health and Disease*. Boca Raton, Fla.: CRC Press.

Pryor, W. A. 1994. "Oxidants and antioxidants." In: *Natural Antioxidants in Human Health and Disease*. Edited by B. Frei. New York: Academy Press, Inc.

Rael, L. T., R. Bar-Or, C. W. Mains, et al. 2009. Plasma oxidation-reduction potential and protein oxidation in traumatic brain injury. *J Neurotrauma* 26, no. 8: 1203–11.

Ragan, D. K., R. McKinstry, T. Benzinger, et al. 2013. Alterations in cerebral oxygen metabolism after traumatic brain injury in children. *J Cereb Blood Flow Metab* 33, no. 1: 48–52.

Rahman, S., K. Bhatia, A. Q. Khan, et al. 2008. Topically applied vitamin E prevents massive cutaneous inflammatory and oxidative stress responses induced by double application of 12-O-tetradecanoylphorbol-13-acetate (TPA) in mice. *Chem Biol Interact* 172, no. 3: 195–205.

Ramlackhansingh, A. F., D. J. Brooks, R. J. Greenwood, et al. 2011. Inflammation after trauma: microglial activation and traumatic brain injury. *Ann Neurol* 70, no. 3: 374–83.

Ramsey, C. P., C. A. Glass, M. B. Montgomery, et al. 2007. Expression of Nrf2 in neurodegenerative diseases. *J Neuropathol Exp Neurol* 66, no. 1: 75–85.

Rao, V. L., M. K. Baskaya, A. Dogan, et al. 1998. Traumatic brain injury down-regulates glial glutamate transporter (GLT-1 and GLAST) proteins in rat brain. *J Neurochem* 70, no. 5: 2020–27.

Rapoport, M. J., S. McCullagh, P. Shammi, et al. 2005. Cognitive impairment associated with major depression following mild and moderate traumatic brain injury. *J Neuropsychiatry Clin Neurosci* 17, no. 1: 61–65.

Ravindran, L. N., and M. B. Stein. 2009. Pharmacotherapy of PTSD: Premises, principles, and priorities. *Brain Res* 1293: 24–39.

Readnower, R. D., J. D. Pandya, M. L. McEwen, et al. 2011. Post-injury administration of the mitochondrial permeability transition pore inhibitor, NIM811, is neuroprotective and improves cognition after traumatic brain injury in rats. *J Neurotrauma* 28, no. 9: 1845–53.

Reger, M. L., A. M. Poulos, F. Buen, et al. 2012. Concussive brain injury enhances fear learning and excitatory processes in the amygdala. *Biol Psychiatry* 71, no. 4: 335–43.

Richardson, J. S. 1993. On the functions of monoamine oxidase, the emotions, and adaptation to stress. *Int J Neurosci* 70, nos. 1–2: 75–84.

Richardson, R., L. Ledgerwood, and J. Cranney. 2004. Facilitation of fear extinction by D-cycloserine: theoretical and clinical implications. *Learn Mem* 11, no. 5: 510–16.

Robertson, C. L., M. J. Bell, P. M. Kochanek, et al. 2001. Increased adenosine in cerebrospinal fluid after severe traumatic brain injury in infants and children: association with severity of injury and excitotoxicity. *Crit Care Med* 29, no. 12: 2287–93.

Robertson, C. L., S. Scafidi, M. C. McKenna, et al. 2009. Mitochondrial mechanisms of cell death and neuroprotection in pediatric ischemic and traumatic brain injury. *Exp Neurol* 218, no. 2: 371–80.

Rosso, I. M., M. R. Weiner, D. J. Crowley, et al. 2013. Insula and anterior cingulate gaba levels in posttraumatic stress disorder: Preliminary findings using magnetic resonance spectroscopy. *Depress Anxiety* 31, no. 2: 115–23.

Rus, H., C. Cudrici, and F. Niculescu. 2005. The role of the complement system in innate immunity. *Immunol Res* 33, no. 2: 103–12.

Ryter, A. 1985. Relationship between ultrastructure and specific functions of macrophages. *Comp Immunol Microbiol Infect Dis* 8, no. 2: 119–33.

Sandhu, J. K., S. Pandey, M. Ribecco-Lutkiewicz, et al. 2003. Molecular mechanisms of glutamate neurotoxicity in mixed cultures of NT2-derived neurons and astrocytes: protective effects of coenzyme Q10. *J Neurosci Res* 72, no. 6: 691–703.

Sano, M., C. Ernesto, and R.G. Thomas et al. 1997. A controlled trial of selegiline, alpha-tocopherol and beta-carotene or both as treatment of Alzheimer's disease. The Alzheimer's Disease Cooperative Study. *N Eng J Med* 336: 1216–22.

Saw, C. L., A. Y. Yang, Y. Guo, et al. 2013. Astaxanthin and omega-3 fatty acids individually and in combination protect against oxidative stress via the Nrf2-ARE pathway. *Food Chem Toxicol* 62: 869–75.

Schelling, G. 2002. Effects of stress hormones on traumatic memory formation and the development of posttraumatic stress disorder in critically ill patients. *Neurobiol Learn Mem* 78, no. 3: 596–609.

Schiavone, S., V. Jaquet, L. Trabace, et al. 2013. Severe life stress and oxidative stress in the brain: from animal models to human pathology. *Antioxid Redox Signal* 18, no. 12: 1475–90.

Schneiderman, A. I., E. R. Braver, and H. K. Kang. 2008. Understanding sequelae of injury mechanisms and mild traumatic brain injury incurred during the conflicts in Iraq and Afghanistan: persistent postconcussive symptoms and posttraumatic stress disorder. *Am J Epidemiol* 167, no. 12: 1446–52.

Schubert, D., H. Kimura, and P. Maher. 1992. Growth factors and vitamin E modify neuronal glutamate toxicity. *Proc Natl Acad Sci USA* 89, no. 17: 8264–67.

Shao, C., K. N. Roberts, W. R. Markesbery, et al. 2006. Oxidative stress in head trauma in aging. *Free Radic Biol Med* 41, no. 1: 77–85.

Sharma, H. S., R. Patnaik, S. Patnaik, et al. 2007. Antibodies to serotonin attenuate closed head injury induced blood brain barrier disruption and brain pathology. *Ann NY Acad Sci* 1122: 295–312.

Sharma, P., B. Benford, Z. Z. Li, et al. 2009. Role of pyruvate dehydrogenase complex in traumatic brain injury and measurement of pyruvate dehydrogenase enzyme by dipstick test. *J Emerg Trauma Shock* 2, no. 2: 67–72.

Shen, W. H., C. Y. Zhang, and G. Y. Zhang. 2003. Antioxidants attenuate reperfusion injury after global brain ischemia through inhibiting nuclear factor-kappa B activity in rats. *Acta Pharmacol Sin* 24, no. 11: 1125–30.

Shohami, E., R. Gallily, R. Mechoulam, et al. 1997. Cytokine production in the brain following closed head injury: dexanabinol (HU-211) is a novel TNF-alpha inhibitor and an effective neuroprotectant. *J Neuroimmunol* 72, no. 2: 169–77.

Shoulson, I. 1998. DATATOP: a decade of neuroprotective inquiry. Parkinson Study Group. Deprenyl And Tocopherol Antioxidative Therapy Of Parkinsonism. *Ann Neurol* 44, no. 3, Suppl 1: S160–66.

Shultz, S. R., F. Bao, V. Omana, et al. 2012. Repeated mild lateral fluid percussion brain injury in the rat causes cumulative long-term behavioral impairments, neuroinflammation, and cortical loss in an animal model of repeated concussion. *J Neurotrauma* 29, no. 2: 281–94.

Singh, I. N., P. G. Sullivan, Y. Deng, et al. 2006. Time course of post-traumatic mitochondrial oxidative damage and dysfunction in a mouse model of focal traumatic brain injury: implications for neuroprotective therapy. *J Cereb Blood Flow Metab* 26, no. 11: 1407–18.

Singh, I. N., P. G. Sullivan, and E. D. Hall. 2007. Peroxynitrite-mediated oxidative damage to brain mitochondria: Protective effects of peroxynitrite scavengers. *J Neurosci Res* 85, no. 10: 2216–23.

Skandsen, T., K. A. Kvistad, O. Solheim, et al. 2010. Prevalence and impact of diffuse axonal injury in patients with moderate and severe head injury: a cohort study of early magnetic resonance imaging findings and 1-year outcome. *J Neurosurg* 113, no. 3: 556–63.

Sonmez, U., A. Sonmez, G. Erbil, et al. 2007. Neuroprotective effects of resveratrol against traumatic brain injury in immature rats. *Neurosci Lett* 420, no. 2: 133–37.

Sproul, T. W., P. C. Cheng, M. L. Dykstra, et al. 2000. A role for MHC class II antigen processing in B cell development. *Int Rev Immunol* 19, nos. 2–3: 139–55.

Steele, M. L., S. Fuller, M. Patel, et al. 2013. Effect of Nrf2 activators on release of glutathione, cysteinylglycine and homocysteine by human U373 astroglial cells. *Redox Biol* 1, no. 1: 441–45.

Stover, J. F., and A. W. Unterberg. 2000. Increased cerebrospinal fluid glutamate and taurine concentrations are associated with traumatic brain edema formation in rats. *Brain Res* 875, nos. 1–2: 51–55.

Stover, J. F., M. C. Morganti-Kosmann, P. M. Lenzlinger, et al. 1999. Glutamate and taurine are increased in ventricular cerebrospinal fluid of severely brain-injured patients. *J Neurotrauma* 16, no. 2: 135–42.

Su, E., M. J. Bell, S. R. Wisniewski, et al. 2010. Alpha-synuclein levels are elevated in cerebrospinal fluid following traumatic brain injury in infants and children: the effect of therapeutic hypothermia. *Dev Neurosci* 32, nos. 5–6: 385–95.

Suh, J. H., S. V. Shenvi, B. M. Dixon, et al. 2004. Decline in transcriptional activity of Nrf2 causes age-related loss of glutathione synthesis, which is reversible with lipoic acid. *Proc Natl Acad Sci USA* 101, no. 10: 3381–86.

Sutherland, A. G., D. A. Alexander, and J. D. Hutchison. 2003. Disturbance of pro-inflammatory cytokines in post-traumatic psychopathology. *Cytokine* 24, no. 5: 219–25.

Suzuki, Y. J., B. B. Aggarwal, and L. Packer. 1992. Alpha-lipoic acid is a potent inhibitor of NF-kappa B activation in human T cells. *Biochem Biophys Res Commun* 189, no. 3: 1709–15.

Tamminga, C., T. Hashimoto, D. W. Volk, et al. 2004. GABA neurons in the human prefrontal cortex. *Am J Psychiatry* 161, no. 10: 1764.

Tavanti, M., M. Battaglini, F. Borgogni, et al. 2012. Evidence of diffuse damage in frontal and occipital cortex in the brain of patients with post-traumatic stress disorder. *Neurol Sci* 33, no. 1: 59–68.

Tavazzi, B., S. Signoretti, G. Lazzarino, et al. 2005. Cerebral oxidative stress and depression of energy metabolism correlate with severity of diffuse brain injury in rats. *Neurosurgery* 56, no. 3: 582–89.

Tavazzi, B., R. Vagnozzi, S. Signoretti, et al. 2007. Temporal window of metabolic brain vulnerability to concussions: oxidative and nitrosative stresses--part II. *Neurosurgery* 61, no. 2: 390–95.

Tezcan, E., M. Atmaca, M. Kuloglu, et al. 2003. Free radicals in patients with post-traumatic stress disorder. *Eur Arch Psychiatry Clin Neurosci* 253, no. 2: 89–91.

Timofeev, I., K. L. Carpenter, J. Nortje, et al. 2011. Cerebral extracellular chemistry and outcome following traumatic brain injury: a microdialysis study of 223 patients. *Brain* 134, Pt 2: 484–94.

Tischler, L., S. R. Brand, K. Stavitsky, et al. 2006. The relationship between hippocampal volume and declarative memory in a population of combat veterans with and without PTSD. *Ann N Y Acad Sci* 1071: 405–9.

Toklu, H. Z., T. Hakan, N. Biber, et al. 2009. The protective effect of alpha lipoic acid against traumatic brain injury in rats. *Free Radic Res* 43, no. 7: 658–67.

Tornwall, M. E., J. Virtamo, P. A. Korhonen, et al. 2004a. Effect of alpha-tocopherol and beta-carotene supplementation on coronary heart disease during the 6-year post-trial follow-up in the ATBC study. *Eur Heart J* 25, no. 13: 1171–78.

Tornwall, M. E., J. Virtamo, P. A. Korhonen, et al. 2004b. Postintervention effect of alpha-tocopherol and beta-carotene on different strokes: a 6-year follow-up of the Alpha Tocopherol, Beta Carotene Cancer Prevention Study, *Stroke* 35, no. 8: 1908–13.

Trembovler, V., E. Beit-Yannai, F. Younis, et al. 1999. Antioxidants attenuate acute toxicity of tumor necrosis factor-alpha induced by brain injury in rat. *J Interferon Cytokine Res* 19, no. 7: 791–95.

Trujillo, J., Y. I. Chirino, E. Molina-Jijon, et al. 2013. Renoprotective effect of the antioxidant curcumin: Recent findings. *Redox Biol* 1, no. 1: 448–56.

Tsuru-Aoyagi, K., M. B. Potts, A. Trivedi, et al. 2009. Glutathione peroxidase activity modulates recovery in the injured immature brain. *Ann Neurol* 65, no. 5: 540–49.

Tyagi, E., R. Agrawal, Y. Zhuang, et al. 2013. Vulnerability imposed by diet and brain trauma for anxiety-like phenotype: implications for post-traumatic stress disorders. *PLoS One* 8, no. 3: e57945.

Vaillancourt, F., H. Fahmi, Q. Shi, et al. 2008. 4-Hydroxynonenal induces apoptosis in human osteoarthritic chondrocytes: the protective role of glutathione-S-transferase. *Arthritis Res Ther* 10, no. 5: R107.

Vaiva, G., V. Boss, F. Ducrocq, et al. 2006. Relationship between posttrauma GABA plasma levels and PTSD at 1-year follow-up. *Am J Psychiatry* 163, no. 8: 1446–48.

van Donkelaar, P., J. Langan, E. Rodriguez, et al. 2005. Attentional deficits in concussion. *Brain Inj* 19, no. 12: 1031–39.

Varma, S., K. L. Janesko, S. R. Wisniewski, et al. 2003. F2-isoprostane and neuron-specific enolase in cerebrospinal fluid after severe traumatic brain injury in infants and children. *J Neurotrauma* 20, no. 8: 781–86.

Vervliet, B. 2008. Learning and memory in conditioned fear extinction: effects of D-cycloserine. *Acta Psychol (Amst)* 127, no. 3: 601–13.

Viano, D. C., E. J. Pellman, C. Withnall, et al. 2006. Concussion in professional football: performance of newer helmets in reconstructed game impacts—Part 13. *Neurosurgery* 59, no. 3: 591–606.

Viano, D. C., I. R. Casson, E. J. Pellman, et al. 2005. Concussion in professional football: comparison with boxing head impacts—Part 10. *Neurosurgery* 57, no. 6: 1154–72.

von Kanel, R., U. Hepp, B. Kraemer, et al. 2007. Evidence for low-grade systemic proinflammatory activity in patients with posttraumatic stress disorder. *J Psychiatr Res* 41, no. 9: 744–52.

Wang, F., Y. H. Li, and Y. L. Hu. 2003. [A study on the expression of C-FOS protein after experimental rat brain concussion]. *Fa Yi Xue Za Zhi* 19, no. 1: 8–9.

Wei, H. H., X. C. Lu, D. A. Shear, et al. 2009. NNZ-2566 treatment inhibits neuroinflammation and pro-inflammatory cytokine expression induced by experimental penetrating ballistic-like brain injury in rats. *J Neuroinflammation* 6: 19.

Wilk, J. E., R. K. Herrell, G. H. Wynn, et al. 2012. Mild traumatic brain injury (concussion), posttraumatic stress disorder, and depression in U.S. soldiers involved in combat deployments: association with postdeployment symptoms. *Psychosom Med* 74, no. 3: 249–57.

Williams, R. W., and K. Herrup. 1988. The control of neuron number. *Annu Rev Neurosci* 11: 423–53.

Woodcock, T., and M. C. Morganti-Kossmann. 2013. The role of markers of inflammation in traumatic brain injury. *Front Neurol* 4: 18.

Wruck, C. J., M. E. Gotz, T. Herdegen, et al. 2008. Kavalactones protect neural cells against amyloid beta peptide-induced neurotoxicity via extracellular signal-regulated kinase 1/2-dependent nuclear factor erythroid 2-related factor 2 activation. *Mol Pharmacol* 73, no. 6: 1785–95.

Wu, A., R. Molteni, Z. Ying, and F. Gomez-Pinilla. 2003. A saturated-fat diet aggravates the outcome of traumatic brain injury on hippocampal plasticity and cognitive function by reducing brain-derived neurotrophic factor. *Neuroscience* 119, no. 2: 365–75.

Wu, A., Z. Ying, and F. Gomez-Pinilla. 2006. Dietary curcumin counteracts the outcome of traumatic brain injury on oxidative stress, synaptic plasticity, and cognition. *Exp Neurol* 197, no. 2: 309–17.

———. 2004. Dietary omega-3 fatty acids normalize BDNF levels, reduce oxidative damage, and counteract learning disability after traumatic brain injury in rats. *J Neurotrauma* 21, no. 10: 1457–67.

————. 2011. The salutary effects of DHA dietary supplementation on cognition, neuroplasticity, and membrane homeostasis after brain trauma. *J Neurotrauma* 28, no. 10: 2113–22.

Wu, Aiguo, Ying Zhe, and F. Gomez-Pinilla. 2010. Vitamin E protects against oxidative damage and learning disability after mild traumatic brain injury in rats. *Neurorehabil Neural Repair* 24, no. 3: 290–8.

Wu, H., A. Mahmood, D. Lu, et al. 2009. Attenuation of astrogliosis and modulation of endothelial growth factor receptor in lipid rafts by simvastatin after traumatic brain injury. *J Neurosurg* 113, no. 3: 591–97.

Xi, Y. D., H. L. Yu, J. Ding, et al. 2012. Flavonoids protect cerebrovascular endothelial cells through Nrf2 and PI3K from beta-amyloid peptide-induced oxidative damage. *Curr Neurovasc Res* 9, no. 1: 32–41.

Xiong, Y., M. Chopp, and C. P. Lee. 2009. Erythropoietin improves brain mitochondrial function in rats after traumatic brain injury. *Neurol Res* 31, no. 5: 496–502.

Xiong, Y., F. S. Shie, J. Zhang, et al. 2005. Prevention of mitochondrial dysfunction in post-traumatic mouse brain by superoxide dismutase. *J Neurochem* 95, no. 3: 732–44.

Xu, Y., B. Ku, L. Cui, et al. 2007. Curcumin reverses impaired hippocampal neurogenesis and increases serotonin receptor 1A mRNA and brain-derived neurotrophic factor expression in chronically stressed rats. *Brain Res* 1162: 9–18.

Yamamoto, T., S. Rossi, M. Stiefel, et al. 1999. CSF and ECF glutamate concentrations in head injured patients. *Acta Neurochir Suppl* 75: 17–19.

Yehuda, R. 2001. Biology of posttraumatic stress disorder. *J Clin Psychiatry* 62, Suppl 17: 41–46.

Yi, J. H., and A. S. Hazell. 2005. N-acetylcysteine attenuates early induction of heme oxygenase-1 following traumatic brain injury. *Brain Res* 1033, no. 1: 13–19.

Yi, J. H., and A. S. Hazell. 2006. Excitotoxic mechanisms and the role of astrocytic glutamate transporters in traumatic brain injury. *Neurochem Int* 48, no. 5: 394–403.

Yi, J. H., R. Hoover, T. K. McIntosh, et al. 2006. Early, transient increase in complexin I and complexin II in the cerebral cortex following traumatic brain injury is attenuated by N-acetylcysteine. *J Neurotrauma* 23, no. 1: 86–96.

Yu, G. F., Y. Q. Jie, A. Wu, et al. 2013. Increased plasma 8-iso-prostaglandin F2alpha concentration in severe human traumatic brain injury. *Clin Chim Acta* 421: 7–11.

Yusuf, S., G. Dagenais, J. Pogue, et al. 2000. Vitamin E supplementation and cardiovascular events in high-risk patients. The Heart Outcomes Prevention Evaluation Study Investigators. *N Eng J Med* 342, no. 3: 154–60.

Zambrano, S., A. J. Blanca, M. V. Ruiz-Armenta, et al. 2013. The renoprotective effect of L-carnitine in hypertensive rats is mediated by modulation of oxidative stress-related gene expression. *Eur J Nutr* 52, no. 6: 1649–59.

Zhang, B., E. J. West, K. C. Van, et al. 2008. HDAC inhibitor increases histone H3 acetylation and reduces microglia inflammatory response following traumatic brain injury in rats. *Brain Res* 1226: 181–91.

Zhu, J., W. Yong, X. Wu, et al. 2008. Anti-inflammatory effect of resveratrol on TNF-alpha-induced MCP-1 expression in adipocytes. *Biochem Biophys Res Commun* 369, no. 2: 471–77.

Zlotnik, A., A. Leibowitz, B. Gurevich, et al. 2012. Effect of estrogens on blood glutamate levels in relation to neurological outcome after TBI in male rats. *Intensive Care Med* 38, no. 1: 137–44.

Zou, Y., B. Hong, L. Fan, et al. 2013. Protective effect of puerarin against beta-amyloid-induced oxidative stress in neuronal cultures from rat hippocampus: involvement of the GSK-3beta/Nrf2 signaling pathway. *Free Radic Res* 47, no. 1: 55–63.

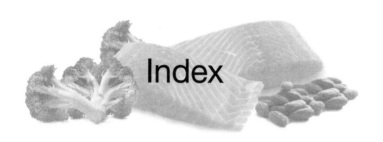

Index

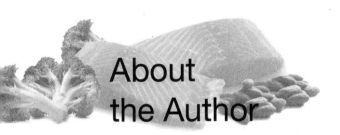

About
the Author

Kedar N. Prasad, Ph.D., former president of the International Society for Nutrition and Cancer, obtained a master's degree in zoology from the University of Bihar, Ranchi, India, and his Ph.D. degree in radiation biology from the University of Iowa, Iowa City, in 1963. He then attended the Brookhaven National Laboratory on Long Island for postdoctoral training before joining the Department of Radiology at the University of Colorado Health Sciences Center, where he became a professor in 1980. Later he was appointed director of the Center for Vitamins and Cancer Research at the University of Colorado School of Medicine. In 1982 he was invited by the Nobel Prize Committee to nominate a candidate for the Nobel Prize in medicine, and in 1999 he was selected to deliver the Harold Harper Lecture at the meeting of the American College of Advancement in Medicine.

His published papers and articles have appeared in such illustrious publications as *Science, Nature,* and *Proceedings of the National Academy of Sciences of the United States of America* (PNAS). He is also the author of several book chapters and twenty-five books, including *Fighting Cancer with Vitamins and Antioxidants.* A member of several professional organizations, he serves as an ad-hoc member of various study sections of the National Institutes of Health (NIH) and has consistently obtained NIH grants for his research.

Kedar N. Prasad is frequently an invited speaker at national and international meetings on nutrition and cancer. He began researching the effects of radiation on animal models in 1963. Over the next thirty-five years, he continued his biological research at three major universities and national research labs, studying the relationships between micronutrients, cancer, and radiation, and focusing on the effects that micronutrients have on human cells and the manner in which they interact with mainstream medical therapies for many common diseases. He found that certain combinations of micronutrients when taken in conjunction with standard treatments, such as chemotherapy, enhanced and complemented the effects of these traditional therapies. The findings inspired him to further his research to determine the effects that these micronutrient combinations might have on other diseases and on general human health.

His present research interests are in the areas of radiation protection, nutrition and cancer, and nutrition and neurological diseases, particularly Alzheimer's disease and Parkinson's disease. He is the former chief scientific officer of the Premier Micronutrient Corporation, which produces antioxidant micronutrient formulations to promote a healthy lifestyle, and he is most recently the chair of the Global Brain Research Institute in Santa Rosa, California.